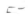

Pau d'Arco

ALSO BY KENNETH JONES:

REISHI: ANCIENT HERB FOR MODERN TIMES
SHIITAKE: THE HEALING MUSHROOM

Pau d'Arco

IMMUNE POWER
FROM THE RAIN FOREST

Kenneth Jones

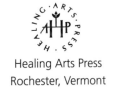

Healing Arts Press
Rochester, Vermont

*To those who risk their life and limb
in the august pursuit of better medicine*

Healing Arts Press
One Park Street
Rochester, Vermont 05767

Note to the reader: *This book is intended as an informational guide. The remedies, approaches, and techniques described herein are meant to supplement, and not to be a substitute for, professional medical care or treatment. They should not be used to treat a serious ailment without prior consultation with a qualified healthcare professional.*

Library of Congress Cataloging-in-Publication Data
Jones, Kenneth, 1954-
    Pau d'arco : immune power from the rain forest / by — 1st ed.
        p. cm.
    Includes bibliographical references and index.
    ISBN 0-89281-497-7
    1. Pau d'arco—Therapeutic use. 2. Tabebuia—Therapeutic use. I. Title.
RM666.P29J66 1993   94-1489
615'.32354—dc20   CIP

Printed and bound in the United States

10   9 8   7   6   5   4   3   2   1

Text design and layout by Leslie Carlson
This book was typeset in Frutiger, with Rodfunk as a display face

Healing Arts Press is a division of Inner Traditions International

Distributed to the book trade in Canada by Publishers Group West (PGW), Toronto,
    Ontario
Distributed to the health food trade in Canada by Alive Books, Toronto and Vancouver
Distributed to the book trade in the United Kingdom by Deep Books, London
Distributed to the book trade in Australia by Millennium Books, Newtown, N. S. W.
Distributed to the book trade in New Zealand by Tandem Press, Auckland

Contents

Acknowledgments

I began this book thirteen years ago, and it grew to occupy most of my spare time. The constraints of personally funding such a lengthy work and the neglect of pau d'arco in medicinal plant research kept it from being completed any sooner. Added to that, most of pau d'arco's uses are centered in South America, which meant that only a few individuals could offer me research assistance. Those who did cut the way across an otherwise insurmountable terrain, the roughest of which was language. I am grateful to Yom Shamash for making invaluable translations of Brazilian studies. Long-awaited, more definitive studies in Germany were expertly translated by Shanti Coble.

Professor Hildebert Wagner and Bernhard Kreher, Ph.D., of the University of Munich and Professor Yoshitsugi Hokama of the University of Hawaii at Manoa are due many warm thanks for keeping me abreast of immunologic assays of pau d'arco. The late Dr. Alwyn H. Gentry, curator of the Missouri Botanical Garden in St. Louis, kindly gave of his precious time whenever I became lost in the botanical maze of *Tabebuia*, the genus to which pau d'arco belongs, and which Gentry had so thoroughly catalogued and clarified shortly before his death. Kenneth Corwin, then of the Herb Exchange in Santa Monica, California; and Teodoro Meyer, Jr., in Tucuman, Argentina, together provided historical and botanical materials that greatly helped me give an accurate account of the medical history of pau d'arco in Argentina and also secured authentic material for the immunologic research that unfolded in Munich and Hawaii.

Thanks are also due to Terrence Mckeena, Ph.D., then at the Department of Botany, University of British Columbia, Vancouver, B.C., Canada, who selflessly offered his expert opinion, and Dennis Awang, Ph.D., then head of the Natural Products Division of the Bureau of Drug Research,

Health and Welfare Canada, in Ottawa, Ontario, Canada, who analyzed pau d'arco from the marketplace along with authentic samples to check for levels of active constituents. Dr. Awang conducted the kind of thorough testing that every popular medicinal plant should receive.

Professor Valter R. Accorsi, a medical botanist at the University of São Paulo, generously shared his experiences with pau d'arco in Brazil. For helpful discussions on Huastec-Mayan uses of the tree in Mexico, I am grateful to Janis B. Alcorn, then at the Department of Botany, University of Texas at Austin, Austin, Texas. Dr. Luis Luna, at the Swedish School of Economics, Helsinki, Finland, generously supplied direct information on the use of pau d'arco from a shaman in the forests of Peru. Dr. Joseph W. Bastien, at the Department of Sociology, Anthropology, and Social Work, University of Texas at Arlington, Arlington, Texas, gave permission to reproduce his photos of Kallaway medicine men and offered useful discussions on folk uses of the tree in Bolivia.

In both South and North America, many people confided to me their experiences with pau d'arco in the treatment of some of the most difficult diseases. For their candor and willingness to discuss conditions of the most private nature, I extend a hearty thanks.

Thanks are also due my publisher, for a job well done and especially to Robin Dutcher-Bayer, whose kind nature helped me to bring this book through its final stages when the work seemed most daunting. Finally, to those closest to me, who were always there to give moral support and encouragement, I offer my eternal thanks.

Introduction

In South America during the 1960s, millions of people's lives were touched with hope and controversy when the media reported that a tea, brewed from the inner bark of a timber tree, was being successfully applied in the treatment of a wide range of diseases, some of them serious. For nearly twenty years afterwards, the use of pau d'arco (pow-darko) *(Tabebuia* spp.) remained largely unknown to all but South Americans. Today, however, the tea is regularly used by at least one million people in North America as well.

The bark of the pau d'arco tree is a traditional folk medicine used in many countries of the tropical Americas. When Europeans arrived in South America they learned herbal medicine from the Indians as a matter of survival in the New World. Since their arrival, use of the bark has been adopted and handed down for generations. Brazilians commonly recall the bark from childhood as something their mothers kept on hand to make tea whenever someone in the family became ill. And, apart from any medicinal purpose, pau d'arco has continued to be enjoyed as a simple refreshment, taken as we would rose hip or some other herbal tea.

In more recent times, pau d'arco has become a source of inspiration for the investigator in search of promising new drugs and the multitude turning to botanical medicines throughout the civilized world. It is my sincere desire that through this book and future efforts, we may one day come to know the major properties of these trees and together gain a deeper understanding of the natural pharmacy growing all around us.

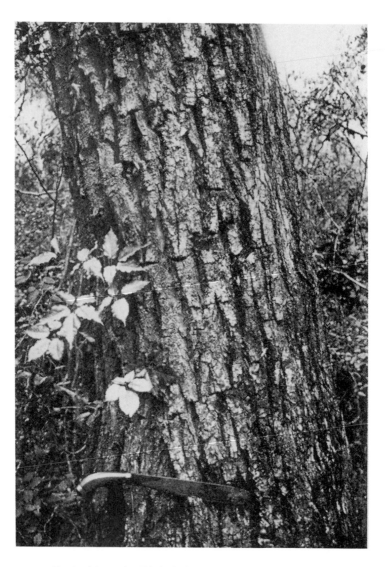

Trunk of Argentine *Tabebuia* showing top leaves of young tree.
From Samuel J. Record and Clayton D. Mell, *Timbers of Tropical America*
(New Haven, Conn.: Yale University Press, 1924), 537.

ONE

A POTION IN THE PRESS

The spring of 1967 found the masses of Brazil reeling from the commotion caused by press reports of a powerful tea made from the bark of the pau d'arco tree. As hundreds offered testimony before the cameras of São Paulo TV, people began ripping the bark from the trees wherever they could be found. A devastation of pau d'arco was seen across the country.[1-4] What with the following announcement in the press, it isn't difficult to see why:

> The story of the discovery is fantastic. But it is nothing compared to the news which could be the most important in the history of humanity: *Cancer has a cure* . . . the news—cure for cancer—is to be taken as being essentially true and honest, or more exactly, strictly scientific.[5]

Strictly speaking, of course, the news was not "scientific" and contrary to what the story would have had people believe, cancer did not at last have a cure. However, key individuals interviewed in that and subsequent reports in the Brazilian news magazine *O'Cruzeiro* have since confirmed that the contents are accurate and represent the only extensive account of pau d'arco's contemporary history in Brazil.

Having traced a seemingly endless number of people who would testify to near-miraculous "cures," *O'Cruzeiro* began with the account of a girl in Rio, sick with cancer, incessantly praying for a cure. In a vision, a monk promised her recovery if she would drink tea brewed from the bark of the pau d'arco tree. But to her parents this was plainly a symptom of her weakened condition and loss of faith in her physicians. In a second visitation, the monk said she would be cured if she drank tea made from the pau d'arco trees growing in Pernambuco or Bahia and then told the news to others. However supernatural, the advice was heeded, and she regained her health.[6] *O'Cruzeiro* learned that from this one case, numerous others had faithfully followed. The trail of cures led to a famous Brazilian herbalist.

THE SKEPTICAL PROFESSOR

Traveling to Piracicaba, the magazine reporters visited the one person who more than any other in Brazil had championed the bark, the botanist Valter Accorsi, professor emeritus at the University of São Paulo. They found him attending lines of over 2,000 people a day. The demand was so great that he worked from dawn to dusk distributing the bark for free.[7] Accorsi began his career in the 1930s and has since accumulated a vast inventory of herbal therapies. He is widely regarded as one of Brazil's most prominent patrons of herbs and is frequently consulted by industry, physicians, and just plain folks, all in search of the knowledge his lifetime with plants provides.[8]

He knew well the episode of the girl in Rio and when close friends started using the bark, he began to study the trees in his own state of São Paulo to see whether they might serve just as well as those from Bahia, located in the northeast of Brazil. He admitted his work could hardly be called scientific; he relied only upon simple observations. The trees from São Paulo in the south had the same qualities, but the northern population from Pernambuco and Bahia seemed best. Taking 400 kilograms from purple- and yellow-flowered pau d'arco, both from Bahia, he compared their effects in leukemia patients. He was convinced that the bark of the purple-flowered pau d'arco was superior.[9]

Accorsi believed he was able to verify "two great truths": The bark eliminated pain and caused a significant increase in the volume of red blood cells. He noted how the bark appeared to be curing everything from diabetes to ulcers and rheumatism, and it seemed to be working in a matter of weeks. Even so, he was reluctant to believe it and for a time kept the information largely to himself.[10]

When the wife of a childhood friend recovered from terminal cancer of the intestine, his innate skepticism finally gave way. Over a period of eight months she had endured five operations. Accorsi explained that after taking the bark she was well again. *O'Cruzeiro* verified the account.[11]

From early in the morning, Accorsi's telephone kept ringing with orders for the bark, mostly from doctors. For the treatment of cancer, he suggested an extract of the bark, a teaspoonful with water at intervals of three hours. Dosages were not exact because, as he explained, the "composition" and levels of active constituents had not been worked out. A dosage limit was regulated with a maximum indicated by the appearance of "a slight rash."[12]

CLINICAL INQUIRY

An interview with Accorsi's sister Gioconda provided leads to more recent cases, and the reporters were suddenly faced with an incredible variety from which to choose. A handful of their verified cases are recounted in the following paragraphs.

A nun with cancer of the tongue finally gave up on conventional treatments when lengthy radiation therapy offered negligible relief and she could no longer talk. Her health restored, she telephoned every week to order the bark for others.[13]

Doctors attending a certain Francisco de Arruda became desperate when they learned their patient had abandoned them to find relief from "Arigo," the famous trance-surgeon who operated with little more than an ordinary pocket-knife.[14] Francisco was found, and the tumor on his scalp was treated with the bark in a topical form. Six years later, when he was ninety-two years old, no sign of the cancer remained.[15]

An oncologist and surgeon, Dr. Jose Iemini related the case of an older man he had previously operated on who should have been dead a year earlier: the cancer was spreading through the stomach and liver. His patient made such a recovery that he was able to visit the clinic by traveling on foot from outside the city.[16]

Dr. Neves was another who was familiar with the bark, but he limited its use mostly to patients with rheumatism. He claimed that the results were "extraordinary." As for cancer, all four of the cases he had treated with pau d'arco were hopeless: "The patients were as old as the cancer."[17]

After seven years of firsthand observation, Accorsi concluded that the bark held six main areas of application: diuretic, sedative, analgesic, decongestant, antibiotic, and cardiotonic.[18]

MEDIA CONFRONTATION

In their follow-up one week later, the *O'Cruzeiro* reporters began dolefully describing the consequences of their first report. Many of the accounts had been supplied by physicians who were now at great risk of losing their licenses by prescribing the bark in hospitals.[19] Another problem was the multitude gathered on the lawns of the hospital at Santo André hoping to obtain the now precious bark. The crowd grew to such a size that the normal function of the hospital was seriously threatened.[20] Here, and at the Hospital of Clinics in São Paulo, signs hung in the hallways announcing that distribution of the bark was suspended.[21] But the public would not be deterred. At the Botanical Gardens in Campinas, then a city of 500,000, and at other reserves across Brazil, droves of people clambered walls and fences to strip the bark from trees conveniently marked as the "purple" pau d'arco by the botanists who tended and now patroled them. Pau d'arco had become a phenomenon.[22]

The reporters confessed that their emphasis on a "cure" for cancer was deliberate, "in order to make [pau d'arco] stand out." They promised to reveal doctors' names, medical histories, X-ray and biopsy test results, and any other documented evidence. But throughout the hospital of Santo André the subject was closed: experiments were stopped,[23] and the entire staff was forbidden to discuss the matter.[24]

Now it was war. Publishing names, incriminating quotations, and, bearing the heading of the hospital, signed prescriptions for the bark in the treatment of cancer and diabetes, *O'Cruzeiro* broke all pacts of silence. The hospital pharmacist, Benedito de Castro, confirmed the studies at the hospital where the bark had always been used and accompanied by a medical prescription. Photographs appeared in *O'Cruzeiro* showing these prescriptions, but de Castro made it known that the hospital was not proclaiming that cancer at last had a cure. His intention was to place a complete dossier in the hands of an authority who after serious investigation would then be able to discuss the subject.[25]

Not everyone was so cautious. Pharmacist Antonio Braga motioned that the bark be acquired for mass distribution to the public. He also felt that the government should take over, and in fact some such efforts were already being made. The Ministry of Agriculture sent samples to the United States, and the federal parliament assigned a commission of inquiry "to clarify what there is to be known."[26]

A meeting was arranged for reporters to put forth further questions at the mayor's office. As the chambers heated with testimony about "cures," the reporters learned that recorded cases of diabetics cured with pau d'arco had gone past the 1,000 mark. Pharmacist Octaviano Gaiarsa recalled cured cases of varicose ulcers, one of anemia, and of skin cancer resistant to all conventional treatments, and one case in which tests had confirmed the remission of osteomyelitis (inflammation of the bone caused by a pus-forming organism). He related the story of "an advanced case of leukemia" that the hospital had assessed as fatal. The white blood cell count was up to 240,000. A month of pau d'arco later, the count was a normal 20,000. Dr. Gaiarsa referred the reporters to the pharmacist de Castro, describing him as very knowledgeable on the subject and one who had compiled a dossier of cases that numbered in the thousands. When de Castro was interviewed he expressed his confidence in the bark, especially against diabetes.[27] (Brazilian scientists have since discovered that like several other Brazilian herbs commonly used to treat diabetes, pau d'arco (*Tabebuia heptaphylla*) inhibits the absorption of glucose in the intestine.[28])

TAKING CONFESSIONS

Another magazine story appeared in June of 1967. The reporters quoted at length from a document jointly prepared by a number of São Paulo physicians. They came forward because they could no longer hold back their "observations and to ask why the medication improves juvenile diabetes in such an impressive manner, reducing the glucose level to the normal amount." (Juvenile diabetes is a severe form of diabetes mellitus that very rarely responds to diet or oral hypoglycemics.) They also wondered, "Why did a cardiac patient at level IV, uncompensated, raised urea, dyspnea, with constant oxygen . . . have complete disappearance of the edema, reduction of urea, and abandon his oxygen bottle at the head of the bed, and return to his activities?" The São Paulo physicians reported that for those suffering incurable disease conditions, pau d'arco "appears to reestablish in them an organic equilibrium, improving even the hematological count."[29]

The news magazine obtained further case histories from a former government health minister, Dr. Sebastien Laet. Despite his admitted perplexity over the bark, he too could not remain silent. Dr. Laet recounted persistent varicose ulcers—over twenty years old—healed in sixteen weeks with an ointment of the bark. Already treated with chemotherapy, a patient suffering terminal breast cancer was not expected to live more than another month. But following the bark treatment for seven months, a biopsy revealed the cancer was gone. A man of eighty-one, semicomatose, urinating profusely, vomiting, and in extreme pain from the cancer in his rectum, should have died. The nurse who attended him recalled the patient they had expected would perish but who was now well.[30]

The São Paulo doctors revealed further instances of ulcers; more remissions from cancer (of the tongue, throat, breast, stomach, and prostate); another cardiovascular disorder; a case of chronic hypertension; and a formerly diabetic physician who claimed to have "cured himself" with the bark. But for the public, confusion soon replaced optimism; the news was just too fantastic. While physicians and patients added corroborating testimony, the São Paulo Hospital of Clinics released a press announcement deriding pau d'arco, saying that the bark provided "no benefit at all for the treatment of cancer." Then from one newspaper to the next, the public didn't know what to believe. One paper cried, "Cures Cancer." Another paper said that the bark "Cures Everything," while in the opposite stream one paper held that pau d'arco "Doesn't Cure Cancer." That paper settled the issue through a simple deduction: pau d'arco was just the annual *cure-all* foisted upon an unfortunate and all too eager public by the unscrupulous. Meanwhile, hucksters began passing off as the *real* pau d'arco barks from at least two other kinds of trees (jaqueira and aroeira trees).[31]

The scientific community had scarcely begun to voice interest. In São Paulo, an independent group of physicians found rats subjected to experimental cancer survived much longer with pau d'arco. And a note on the bark in *Pulso*, a journal from the Winthrop Laboratories in Brazil, reported that a Professor Italo Boquino and colleagues had found activity against diabetes and gastritis.[32] There was *something* to the folk remedy, after all. But how much was anyone's guess.

From the day *O'Cruzeiro's* first story appeared on the newsstands in Brazil, pau d'arco was never again prescribed at the Hospital of Santo André, at least not so openly. The bark was not approved as a drug for the treatment of any condition, and so legally its prescription was out of the question. More than twenty years later, questions about *how* pau d'arco works continue to be raised, and I expect that to continue for years to come. On two occasions since 1967, a new clinical director at the hospital, Dr. Fadlo Fraige Filho, had made concerted efforts to conduct a full "scientific study" of patients on the bark. Once in 1975 and again in 1979, he tried to encourage the cooperation of his fellow physicians. But each time the voting majority of doctors at the hospital declined: they would have nothing to do with such a scheme for fear of being labeled *quacks*.[33]

ELIXIR FOR THE ARGENTINES

Pau d'arco next became front page news in Argentina's northwest in October 1967. An article in the newspaper *Ultima Linea* revealed that in the city of San Miguel de Tucuman, located at the foothills of the Andes, a tea, salve, and extract of a bark from local timbers was being applied in the treatment of asthma, cancer, eczema, leukemia, and rheumatism. Early records held that it "acted like a tonic" and wakened the appetite. Yet doctors were seeing changes they couldn't explain.[34]

The bark would also have a mentor in Argentina. A colleague of Professor Accorsi, Teodoro Meyer[35] (1911–72) served as professor of botany

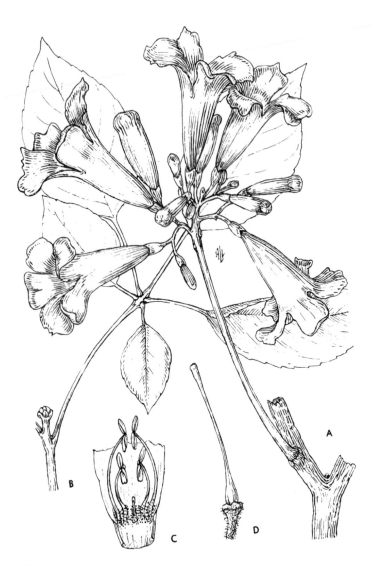

Tabebuia avellanedae Lor. ex Griseb. From Antonio P. L. Digilio and Pablo R. Legname, *Los Arbols Indigenas de la Provincia de Tucuman, Opera Lilloana XV* (Tucuman, Argentina: National University of Tucuman, 1966), IOI.

and plant geography at the Miguel Lillo Institute and Herbarium in San Miguel de Tucuman.[36] From there he was a principal supplier of herbs to pharmaceutical companies in search of new agents to combat disease. For example, he provided the drug giant Merck and Co. of New Jersey with herbs used in folk medicine to treat fevers and malaria.[37] According to his son, medicinal plants had been his father's greatest love ever since he was a young man. He spoke Spanish and German, but, more important, he had learned the tongue of the local Indians and so had access to their knowledge of medicinal plants.[38] He was also a distinguished botanist.[39] In 1965 he received Argentina's first National Prize in Biology for his contributions to the field.[40]

During his study of pau d'arco, Meyer kept in touch with Accorsi in Brazil while extending his own investigations to include closely related trees in countries adjacent to Argentina. Local biochemists assisted him in developing an "alcohol-free fluid extract" that he called an "elixir."[41] He formulated this elixir from the inner barks of three kinds of pau d'arco growing in Argentina, where they are called lapacho trees. From the northwest, he gathered the barks of *Tecoma fabrisi* Meyer[42] (one he described and named for science)[43] and lapacho rosado (*Tabebuia avellanedae* Lorentz = *Tabebuia impetiginosa*).[44] The third bark, the lapacho morado (*Tabebuia ipé* Mart. = *Tabebuia heptaphylla*), came from Corrientes Province in the northeast.[45]

His instructions for preparing the "tea" called for ten grams of bark (about six tablespoons) to four cups of boiling water (see also "Preparation and Dosage," page 13). He boiled the bark until the water was reduced to three cups (about five minutes) and then let it cool.[46] Meyer further instructed as follows:

> Let it cool and then filter it through a piece of cloth. Give it to the patient during the day. It is preferable to give the patient one cup during the morning, one at midday, and the last before dinner time. Take it cold, warm, or hot without sugar. Prepare the liquid in the morning and keep it in the refrigerator throughout the day. Drink it without interruption but don't drink it too quickly.[47]

In the treatment of "grave cases," his instructions to the physician

were to use the tea in combination with the extract, alternating throughout the day, ". . . one spoonful of elixir three times a day, besides the
three cups of Lapacho, spacing them every three hours."[48] Meyer also
left the following advice:

> In the treatment of "incurable" diseases such as cancer and leukemia,
> the treatment will be very lengthy and in most cases, for the rest of the
> patient's life. It is noteworthy when a few months of such treatment suc-
> ceeds in controlling, reducing and stabilizing the illness. Even when analyti-
> cal data support a negative diagnosis (i.e., the apparent absence of the
> disease), one should not trust these results, for the symptoms and pains will
> return some time after stopping treatment . . . the explanation lies in the
> fact that such illnesses are typically discovered in an advanced stage; better
> results could be expected if treatment were started near the onset of the
> malady.
>   To sum up, the treatment of "incurable" illnesses must be lengthy, un-
> interrupted and maintained at a minimum useful dosage."[49]

Meyer began this work knowing only that the bark was used by the
Indians "for healing and revitalizing." To find cancer patients in the last
stages of disease suffering so little pain on the bark that they had no
need for sedatives was something completely unexpected. But what he
had witnessed he couldn't deny; he saw a noticeable improvement in
both their "general state and their spirits."[50]

In the spring of 1966 he urged the University of Tucuman to begin a
full investigation. This was denied on two very common grounds: a lack
of equipment and the all too familiar lack of funds. About a year later
Ultima Linea reported the sensational story of Dr. Meyer and the people
of Tucuman who were curing diseases with the bark. As word of the
cures spread from one news service and then one country to the next,[51]
Meyer found a deluge of mail impossible to answer.[52] Finally, he turned
to physicians in Argentina who would share their own findings with him
about the results obtained with their patients,[53] and he sent the bark to
their clinics across the country.[54]

There was nothing illegal in his dispensing the extract, but by the
spring of 1969 the Medical College made certain it was banned—an act
that prompted public disdain. Immediately after, a letter from a local citi-

zen protesting the action appeared in *La Gazeta*, the most conservative paper in the province. It was typical of many others received.[55] Pointing up Meyer's background as "not just some quack or healer," the letter stated it seemed the ban was part of a plan by the medical profession to keep Argentina's large population down. The writer went on to say how such a ban would not have occurred in the United States or any other country, where, instead of rebuke, Meyer would have received collaborative support in his study of an agent "that attacks the nightmare of the twentieth century."[56]

Meyer maintained his scientific composure just the same. No matter the number of cases in his own country and those constant reports from Brazil, *Ultima Linea* found him "reluctant to say that cancer is cured because of Lapacho."[57] But this was of no consequence to the Medical College. Should he persist in dispensing his elixir, a fund awarded as part of the National Prize in Biology four years earlier, which he had hoped to spend on studies of the bark, was now threatened with being revoked. This event destroyed his faith in a fraternity of which he had for so long been a part. Teodoro Meyer died soon after and is fondly remembered by the people of Tucuman to this day.[58]

PREPARATION AND DOSAGE

The usual procedure for making the tea is to boil water, let it cool to hot, add the bark, and allow it to simmer for twenty minutes. The amount of bark to use varies from one authority to the next, with two tablespoons of bark to three cups of water about average. The number of grams that make up a tablespoon varies somewhat from one brand name to the next, but six tablespoons of bark equaling ten grams is common. In addition to the loose tea form, the bark is widely available in South and North American health food stores in the form of a fluid extract under various brand names.

Some have boiled the bark for five or as long as twenty minutes before letting it simmer. Others have let it boil for a full hour. The advantage or disadvantage of this remains to be studied. As for cooking ware, Pyrex is ideal. Aluminum is not advised. Several of my informants have stressed a further precaution, in that contact of the tea or extract with plastics seems to negate desired effects, although this too remains to be investigated.

From a pharmacist referred to me by Professor Accorsi, the dosage of bark tea in Brazil is three to six "teacups" per day, with "large amounts" in serious diseases. The tea is prepared by placing four teaspoons of bark in one pint of water, which is brought to a boil and left to simmer for fifteen minutes. For serious illnesses, the bark extract is taken with water, one teaspoonful to a half glass per hour, or every two and three hours for less serious cases and for regular use, respectively. In any application, the tea is recommended for use along with the extract.[59]

TWO

PAU D'ARCO IN THE NORTH

The science of ethnobotany was described in the last century as the examination of "plants used by primitive and aboriginal people."[1] In 1967 Richard Schultes of Harvard University gave a more encompassing description: "The relationships between man and his ambient vegetation."[2] Use of pau d'arco outside of the area it grows in is technically the subject of economic botany, which studies "*indirect* contact with the plants through their by-products."[3] But by studying the uses of a plant or its by-products in another culture, the ethnobotanist may obtain a far greater understanding of potential applications for a plant in any culture. The arena of medical uses brings in the ethnopharmacologist, who will look very carefully at cross-cultural uses, for these are important clues to pharmacologic activity: the more separated two cultures or tribes that utilize a plant for the same purposes, the greater the chances that plant will have measurable activity against a disease instead of being just another nostrum, or quack remedy. I found few uses for pau d'arco not employed in the tropical Americas.

In our contemporary folk medicine, pau d'arco is today very much a part of the home medicine chest. In the United States, where the bark has been available for over ten years now, pau d'arco continues to inspire testimonies from formerly ill individuals who often tried the herb when all else had failed. It is also significant to note that these applications of pau d'arco include many uses found in the tropical Americas that were not known to the North Americans who tried them.

When in Canada pau d'arco became widely reputed as an alternative treatment for cancer, the Health Protection Branch of the federal government (Canada's Food and Drug Administration) classified the bark as a "new drug." For a time, this effectively banned its sale, but not without protest. In the East, crowds demonstrated in front of the Parliament building in the nation's capital. In the West, at the U.S./Canada border near Vancouver, the six-o'clock news panned protestors decked in Boston Tea Party garb waving placards and shouting "Free the tea!" The government edict still stands, but I have yet to find a health food or herb store in Canada that today doesn't carry the bark.

Pau d'arco finally reached the United States in 1981. It all began with a newspaper article highlighting the news from *O'Cruzeiro* in the 1960s.[4] In the same year, one botanist announced that the bark was "threatening to become a second laetrile."[5] At the time, he made no exaggeration. In one of the earliest voices of the laetrile therapy, the *Cancer News Journal*, author and herbalist Louise Tenney provided many examples of Americans with cancer in remission after they drank the tea.[6-8] In 1983, a Florida writer traced accounts extending from the Caribbean to Canada. In Houston a woman had used the bark to treat diabetes. She was able to reduce her insulin dosage by 50 percent and her average blood sugar level dropped by more than half. A doctor in Fort Lauderdale had several patients "saved" from cancer, a woman in Illinois was in remission from skin cancer, and a nurse in New Jersey had provided the bark to three diabetics. The nurse reported that after seventy-two hours all three had found they could reduce their insulin intake by half, just like the woman in Houston.[9]

Meanwhile, in the Canadian press, it was reported that a physician had told a leukemia patient using pau d'arco that he didn't want to know what it was his patient was taking, but thought it should probably be continued.[10] In 1985 in Vancouver, a major daily interviewed a man who had refused treatment for a cancerous tumor in his throat. When later he started on pau d'arco, he found the pain "lessened considerably," and his physician confirmed the cancer was diminishing.[11] I came across another case in a farming area east of Vancouver that didn't make the press. It involved a young man in his early twenties with a brain tumor diagnosed as rapidly spreading glioblastoma. He was given radiation treatment, but eventually his body wouldn't tolerate any more, and the tumor continued to grow. He wasn't expected to live for more than another two months. After several liters of the tea daily for a week, he started to feel better, and in another month no sign of the tumor could be found. Soon after, he was assessed fit and healthy enough to continue his service in the Canadian Armed Forces. In a similar case of a young woman in the same farming district, the obstruction was not clearly diagnosed as a tumor and the patient had not received any other treatment.

I wondered whether accounts of cancer remissions would eventually fade away, but in 1993 two more cases were reported in the United States,[12] indicating there are other accounts of remissions not receiving attention. Even so, pau d'arco is not a sure cure for cancer. In fact, in Brazil one pharmacist referred to me by Professor Accorsi lists the bark extract only as "auxiliary in fighting neoplasia."[13]

The cases are endless, and I am certain book after book could be written on case histories alone. The various kinds of conditions treated here are at least as diverse as those in South America during the 1960s. These are anecdotal accounts and to most physicians are considered worthless of follow-up. How often these accounts were the result of a placebo response no one, of course, knows. But for the ethnobotanist in search of promising herbs in folk medicine, the accounts carry the same weight as those from the Indians in the rain forests. On the basis of congruent uses, plants become more promising candidates for the pharmaco-botanist to investigate than plants with consistently different uses from one group of people to the next, for, as mentioned earlier, when people in separate areas of the world utilize the same herb for the same ailments, the ethnobotanist is more assured that the plant-medicine in question may hold activity against the particular ailments treated. To give you an example, a pharmaceutical attorney informed me that since drinking this "jungle-juice," the cataracts he couldn't get rid of have gone and he no longer needs thyroid medication. He was originally drinking the tea in an attempt to relieve a persistent flu. An ethnobotanist would then check the recorded uses of pau d'arco to see whether indigenous people had used the bark for thyroid problems, cataracts, or eye ailments.

In the contemporary folk medicine of North America, other conditions the "natives" here are treating include sinusitis and, using the tea as a mouthwash, stubborn gum diseases. From bathing their eyes with the tea, a number of people have told me their cataracts dissolved. In emphysema, some experimenters believe inhaling the vapor from the hot tea is especially beneficial. There are also individuals who claim that for circulation problems and migraine headaches, the tea alone was of benefit. One man I spoke with suffered for over twenty years with migraines, but since drinking the tea, he claims the headaches have not returned. In a similar application, a man who had recently endured five major surgical operations told me he found immediate relief from the side-effect of day-to-day hemorrhaging after only a few cups of the tea. After the problem had long since gone, he insisted on drinking pau d'arco daily.

A number of regular users mentioned that the bark sometimes affects the bowels by loosening the stool. This seems to be a consistent experience from using large amounts of pau d'arco—usually, liters per day. Then again, one of my informants related an incident in which a child who had chronic diarrhea and was resistant to all manner of treatment finally recovered after the parents administered only half a cup of the tea. I also interviewed a woman who had practically the reverse situation: She told me that ten years earlier she had suffered from an obstruction of the bowels and they had failed to function properly since. An operation removed nineteen inches of bowel, but she still had cramps and the nuisance of regular constipation. Her only recourse at the time was suppositories and a wide assortment of laxatives. The change after using pau d'arco was dramatic. She claimed that within one week on the tea the problem was gone—without any suppositories or laxatives.

Naturopathic physicians, who practice medicine using heat, water, diet, and other "drugless" therapies, have taken special notice. They have recommended pau d'arco to patients with yeast infections and skin problems, such as acne, pimples, psoriasis, and rashes. A cream has been used to treat sunburn, and a simple homemade ointment consisting of finely powdered bark in a lanolin base has been used to provide pain relief and to speed the mending of wounds. Bark ointments are used against burns, common skin rash, cuts, cysts, and hemorrhoids.

I found more than one instance in which shingles, a disease caused by *Herpes zoster*, was treated with the tea by frequent sponging of the sores and taking the tea internally along with a bark extract. Daily treatment periods of eight hours or more lasting three weeks obviously required great perseverance. These individuals claimed no other medication was employed except for a light vegetable oil applied before bedtime to prevent the skin from cracking. One doctor I related this account to said, "You would think these people were living in the third world!" But it wasn't the money: they had simply given up on conventional medicine after experiencing side-effects and gaining no significant relief from their problems.

Another instance of external application involved an outpatient with extensive third-degree burns to the torso. The tea was applied topically by frequent sponging, and it was also taken internally. Photographs documenting the treatment showed a rapid and remarkable recovery, with the patient claiming relief from unbearable pain after the very first application.

Burns, hemorrhoids, cuts, cysts, skin eruptions, and rashes are all reminiscent of the various external applications of pau d'arco bark teas and decoctions made in the rain forests of tropical America, a subject we'll explore in the next chapter. Much of the success of these applications is undoubtedly owed in large part to tannins and related substances (flavonoids) found in the bark of pau d'arco and many other trees. I know many people will find the use of pau d'arco in the treatment of third-degree burns too much to believe, and I concur that the report needs clinical study for verification. But that wouldn't be the only time such an application has occurred.

An important example of a bark being used for treating burns that is reminiscent of this use of pau d'arco was found in Mexico in 1982. The finely powdered inner bark of a Mexican tree called tepeschuite (*Mimosa tenuiflora* [Willd.] Poiret) was successfully applied to burn victims of a natural gas explosion at San Juanica, Mexico City. Besides treating burns, folk-medical use of the bark includes the prevention of inflammation. The bark of tepeschuite, which contains a "great amount" of tannins, was used again in 1985 when the city was struck with an earthquake. Numerous scientists and reporters from all over the world witnessed the results of this treatment, finding a pain-relieving effect that lasted as long as three hours and complete healing of the skin in a matter of several weeks. The bark powder was also credited with a significant reduction in the death rate from more severe burns.[14]

As a result of all the media attention, tepeschuite is now being collected for the manufacture of creams designed for skin repair and skin protection and recovery from sunburn. European dermatologists have found the bark extract inhibits free radicals, improves the microcirculation of the skin, and increases the damage resistance of small blood vessels.[15] This plant grows in southeast Mexico in the Cintalapa Valley in the state of Chiapas, where for hundreds if not thousands of years, the "skin tree" has efficiently served as a remedy for burns and inflammation of the skin.[16] One would think this common name alone would have been enough of a lead to tempt investigation, but, as is often the case, we Westerners are slow to regard anything so primitive.[17]

There are other similarities of the skin tree to pau d'arco. As with pau d'arco, the bark of the skin tree is first subjected to fire until hardened and then powdered for sprinkling on burns and lesions. Remarkably, even after the heat of a direct flame, the bark (in a water or alcoholic extract) retains significant antimicrobial activity against such difficult pathogens as *Candida albicans* and *E. coli* (*Escherichia coli*), and especially staph (*Staphylococcus aureus*), for which the bark showed an inhibitory activity comparable to the antibiotic streptomycin.[18] *Candida albicans* and *S. aureus* are far more toxic in a combined infection, each contributing to infection by the other. To give you some idea of *how* toxic this combination of pathogens can be, infection by either organism alone in mice caused no fatalities, but in the same doses the two combined caused every mouse to die. In other words, these pathogens are synergistically toxic.[19] A simple extract made by boiling the bark of a pau d'arco (*Tabebuia impetiginosa*) from northwest Argentina was recently found to display high activity against a penicillin G–resistant strain of *Staphylococcus aureus*. Curiously enough, the bark of a pau d'arco from the northeast of Argentina (*Tabebuia heptaphylla* [Vell.] Toledo) was without antimicrobial activity (against *E. coli*, penicillin G–resistant *S. aureus*, and *Aspergillus niger*).[20]

For burns, tannic acid was itself once the preferred treatment. In 1929 the Medical Council of Great Britain hailed that treatment for reducing burn mortalities by over 30 percent, eliminating or decreasing shock and acute toxemia, and greatly reducing or eliminating pain after "the first few applications." In the medical therapeutics of the day, the tannic acid treatment for burns was praised as "one of the most important recent advances."[21] In Germany, owing to the war, tannic acid treatment of burns continued until 1948, long after British and American doctors had abandoned it because of liver toxicity. Tannic acid is absorbed through the skin and then travels directly to the liver. Because of the large amounts required in burn therapy, liver necrosis was killing patients at the same time the treatment dramatically healed their burns.[22]

Owing to the relatively small amounts of tannin in teas as compared to the tannic acid treatment of burns, one could expect that liver toxicity would be minimized; however, where large areas of the body are involved and the treatment is lengthy, there is obviously some reason for caution in using any tannin-containing tea for burns.

The bottom line here is that unlike some "new drug," pau d'arco has not undergone the rigors of clinical trials, and we therefore do not know how effective or noneffective it would be in the treatment of any disease. Until such a time, ascribing even so much as a temporary remission to the bark will be met with extreme skepticism. In the meantime, the "natives" continue to experiment.

ALLERGY SYNDROMES

One of the most popular uses for pau d'arco in North America has been the treatment of so-called *allergy syndromes*. Again, patients self-medicating with the bark were typically those who found little or no relief from conventional prescriptions and were often experiencing side effects.[23] Frequently, those using the bark are people who suffer from reactions to yeasts and molds, and especially to *Candida albicans*, a common fungus or "yeast" found in humans and animals that some physicians suspect is the underlying cause of food allergies, extreme sensitivity to chemicals in the environment, and disorders of the immune system.[24–28]

One of what would eventually be many articles on this subject appeared in the popular health magazine *Let's Live* in February 1984. Titled "*Candida albicans*: A Lingering Problem," the article by Robert E. Foreman, Ph.D., described the symptoms as a "bewildering array," with more than one occurring at the same time. Popularly known as candidiasis, this syndrome offers a horrific range of symptoms with about as many combinations as there are possible problems with an automobile. Foreman listed arthritis, asthma, cystitis, migraine and other headaches, immobility of the joints, gas and bloating, spastic colitis, oral thrush, lesions and skin rashes, and irregular bowel movements "ranging from severe chronic constipation . . . to frequent (as many as 15 per day) loose and sometimes uncontrolled movements." He added lethargy, "hormonal irregularities," chronic muscle pains, and a variety of mental and emotional states such as anxiety, depression (extremely common), poor memory, irritability, "and even cases diagnosed as schizophrenia."[29]

Currently, a diagnosis of chronic fatigue syndrome might replace a previous diagnosis of yeast syndrome for many.[30–34] It is interesting to note that today there are herbal formulas containing pau d'arco used in chronic fatigue and in allergies.[35] One authority on yeast syndrome, William G. Crook, M.D., observes that many chronic fatigue syndrome patients have shown rapid improvement following treatment for yeast infections.[36]

As with chronic fatigue syndrome, the main problem has been a consensus of diagnosis.[37] Partly due to *Candida*'s wide distribution in the body, tests have offered little accuracy. And while some promising work in developing tests that are accurate provides hope,[38,39] there are reports that when patients suspected of having yeast syndrome are treated as though they do (regardless of test results to the contrary), many of them have experienced dramatic improvement.[40] The most promising and accurate test for Candida complex available today is the CandiSphere Enzyme Immunoassay test (CEIA), which has shown a diagnostic accuracy of 92 percent.[41] Because in the past the confirmation or the rejection of the diagnosis has largely depended on patient response and nonresponse to anticandidiasis treatment, the would-be patient should seek a physician already familiar with the symptoms.[42–46]

Yeast syndrome has become widely known, and it appears epidemic in proportion. Some frightening allergy states, such as "total allergy syndrome," have been suspected as stemming from the same fungus. With this syndrome one becomes allergic to practically everything. Doctors who deal with these states, called "clinical ecologists," have not been in agreement about either the cause or how many people may be affected. The clinical ecologist often points to *accumulated poisoning from a chemically overburdened environment weakening our body's defense systems.*[47–49] The same syndrome is now called twentieth-century disease, multiple-chemical sensitivity (MCS),[50] and environmental illness (EI).[51] Seventy to 80 percent of the patients with this syndrome are women, but no one knows why.[52] In the early 1970s the same symptoms matched those of "allergic tension-fatigue syndrome" and 72 percent of those affected were women. The most frequently reported symptom was "fatigue" (94 percent), and food "sensitivities" affected 91 percent.[53] Today, at least 90 percent of the symptoms are also reported in chronic fatigue syndrome.[54] A partial list of symptoms follows:[55]

asthma	skin rashes
fatigue	migraines
blurred vision	heart pounding
short-term memory loss	earaches
shortness of breath	dizziness
learning disabilities	depression
spaciness	clumsiness
cold intolerance	indigestion
backaches	hypersensitivity to molds
"immune system dysregulation"	headaches

alcohol intolerance	joint pains/muscle pains
nasal stuffiness	frequent colds
sleepiness	bloating
spasms	constipation/diarrhea

On the fungal side are studies in animals showing that *Candida* toxins—by-products of the original fungus created within the system—can produce many of the symptoms commonly associated with the allergy-to-everything syndrome. Gail Nielsen of the Candida Research and Information Foundation in Castro Valley, California, explains that the symptoms produced by these toxins are severe. They include "paralysis of the extremities, lesions in various organs, edema and changes in the cerebrum, and, in some cases, even death."[56]

Blaming pollution, clinical ecologists maintain that even minute amounts of certain chemicals in our foods and "environment" can be the cause of mental and physical problems.[57] A report by the U.S. National Research Council costing $2.2 million undoubtedly confirmed some of their worst suspicions. Incredibly, the three-year study found "no toxicity information exists for nearly 80 percent of the chemicals used in commercial products and processes." Of over 67,000 different chemicals, the list included "no toxicity data available" for 25 percent of drugs and "inert" substances used in their formulation; 48 percent of food additives; 56 percent of ingredients used in cosmetics; and from 76 to 82 percent of other commercial chemicals.[58] With so little testing it is fair to conclude that the potential exists for human poisoning on a massive scale—to say nothing of what all those substances may be doing in various combinations.

The director of occupational medicine at Yale University, Mark Cullen, M.D., and other academic and state medical authorities in the United States and Canada have recognized the EI diagnosis as valid.[59] However, the very existence of EI has been questioned by others: many physicians are typically concerned that patients with psychiatric illnesses are being mistreated.[60, 61] The Environmental Protection Agency (EPA) not only recommends more research of EI, it is now also pursuing such research, along with the National Academy of Sciences.[62]

Allergists are currently seeing an increasing number of patients who can no longer wear fabrics made of synthetics, eat produce from the supermarket, drink water from the tap, handle a newspaper, use ordinary detergents and cleansers, and in some cases even breathe without a gas mask.[63] Whatever the cause, the body's inability to defend itself against *Candida* has been suspected to underlie all these sensitivities.[64,65]

THE PAU D'ARCO TREATMENT

Several popular books note the use of pau d'arco against yeast syndrome.[66] One authority on herbal medicine in America, Michael A. Weiner, Ph.D., found that hundreds of U.S. physicians have attested to pau d'arco's use against this syndrome and that its efficacy is backed by approximately one million patients regularly applying the tea.[67]

The possibility of pau d'arco as an alternative remedy against allergies and yeast syndrome first came to light in 1983. Gail Nielsen was one of the earliest experimenters, and she eventually began a newsletter on the syndrome that would provide much needed information for the physician and for others suffering the same dilemma.[68] Her own case is apparently not uncommon.[69] She was acutely sensitive to chemicals and mold. The incapacitating cerebral difficulties kept her homebound for more than a year.[70] Medication was an antifungal agent called nystatin, taken in pill form, sixteen a day.[71] She was a year on pau d'arco tea and maintaining a diet low in carbohydrates before going off the antifungal without difficulty, and in another six months she began to live normally. She noticed her severe reactions to mold greatly diminished after only one month on the tea, a few cups a day at most.[72-74]

Nielsen's notes, including the findings of fellow sufferers and physicians, contain many fascinating observations. For example, it seems that some people can't tolerate the tea without allergiclike reactions and that for many certain brands have not been "well tolerated," especially by those who have "chemical" sensitivities. Others have found they can work up to taking the tea full strength by first taking it diluted (as little as a drop or two per liter of water) and then over a period of weeks or even months, gradually increasing the strength.[75] She found patients usually started with half to a full cup a day, increasing consumption to a "maintenance" dosage of four per day over a period of about four weeks. For some, a longer time was needed to reach maintenance.[76] She and others have found that what seems to happen to yeast syndrome patients on the bark is a temporary reversal and regression of symptoms. Nielsen writes:

> All have shared with me experiences of going back through old symptoms. Many of these we all have in common, while some are peculiar to the individual . . . users reveal that their reexperienced symptoms appear suddenly, stay for varying lengths of time, then disappear."[77]

The current hypothesis has it that these reexperienced symptoms, which last for short periods, occur as the yeast dies off; filtering through the blood system, the dead cells cause allergiclike reactions.[78] These reactions might occur after taking *any* agent that fights the fungus.

After six years of observation, Nielsen reported that patients on the tea told of suddenly finding themselves more resilient to chemicals, foods, and molds. And while still having symptoms of the syndrome, they claimed a greater sense of well-being, both physically and mentally. Others reported skin rashes clearing, as well as fungus of the nails, and several patients found the tea highly effective as a douche against vaginal yeast infection.[79]

A doctor in Mill Valley, California, saw one patient with a "difficult case of vaginal yeast" that cleared up in only two hours with this method.[80] I spoke with several physicians in the eastern United States who related nearly identical cases. They told me that most of their patients were experiencing allergic reactions to prescription and some nonprescription medications they had tried, and, except for the douche with pau d'arco, they were not having any success against the problem. These observations obviously merit clinical research.

Nielsen is careful to point out that the path to recovery requires enormous perseverance and that not everyone claims relief, no matter what the medication.[81] She notes that "one patient reported feeling better when off it."[82] Those who have experienced improvement explained it was a gradual process, usually taking many months.

LETHAL CONNECTIONS

Yeast infection is not limited to those who are simply "allergic."[83, 84] It extends to include those with immunodeficiencies, diabetes mellitus, lymphoma, and leukemia and people who have undergone treatments with immunosuppressive drugs, antibacterial antimicrobics, glucosteroids, or birth control pills. Studies have found that intravenous catheters, antibiotics, chemotherapy, and high sugar levels in the blood are common conditions preceding widespread internal infection by *Candida*.[85–87] The anti-*Candida* drug nystatin was not significantly effective in those who had antibiotic as well as chemotherapy treatments.[88]

A symposium on candidiasis in 1983 heard the chairperson, Gerald P. Bodey, M.D., from the M.D. Anderson Hospital and Tumor Institute in Houston, remark at the current increase in early fungal infections seen in acute leukemia. In one population of leukemia patients being treated with their first chemotherapy, 58 percent had successful treatment, finding complete remission. However, among those who perished with leukemia, 71 percent died from "infections complication." Of those, 40 percent died because of fungal infection.[89] Infections also caused more deaths in cases of solid tumors.[90]

Candida is among the more common pathogenic fungi causing infections in patients with low counts of neutrophils—an immune system cell that eats foreign and pathogenic intruders. In cancer patients with defective T-lymphocytes (T-cells), *Candida* is again among the most common infecting entities.[91] The situation for the cancer patient is made all the worse by a fungal infection. Researchers at the Mayo Clinic in Rochester, Minnesota, found that patients with fungal infection, whether disseminated or even localized, show a dysfunctional T-cell reactivity to foreign cells: the numbers of T-cells may be normal, but their immunologic activity is suppressed.[92]

The subjects of yeast syndrome, chronic fatigue syndrome and environmental illness—all showing many symptoms in common—can scarcely be covered in the few pages here. And while a vast and growing amount of literature suggests an assortment of remedies to try, I must emphasize that physicians familiar with these syndromes should be consulted first.

Very often, these are physicians who practice "preventive" medicine. But regardless of the kind of shingle they hang, the care and monitoring doctors can provide may be invaluable.

WHY PAU D'ARCO?

As pau d'arco's history emerged, the bark became popularly regarded as a stimulant and restorer of the immune system, even without the public having the assurance of studies to show such activity. Many believe pau d'arco to be particularly valuable in managing allergies, including those associated with yeast syndrome.

Indications of an immunologic basis to the yeast syndrome continued to mount until 1985, when clinical ecologists of the American Academy of Environmental Medicine provided the name *immune system dysregulation* (ISD). This new term encompassed both the rapid and gradual immunologic malfunction that *Candida* toxins are known to induce. With ISD, which some now believe to be identical with chronic fatigue syndrome,[93] the allergic responses to *Candida* and other common allergens result from what is regarded as a previously overlooked problem with the immune system. In other words, ISD seems to differ from what allergists have for so long been seeing in patients who have "allergies" in the way the immune system malfunctions. T-cells have been the main suspects. When their population decreases or their functional ability becomes hampered, the antibody-forming B-cells that they regulate have a more difficult time distinguishing the harmful effects of toxic substances from harmless substances entering the body.[94] That would also apply to CFS patients, who, coincidentally or not, have a high incidence of allergies.[95]

Patients with recurrent vaginitis caused by *C. albicans* have been found with a lymphocyte suppressor, the production of which appears to be induced by the fungus. This immunosuppressant then blocks the immune system (lymphocytes) from fully responding to the fungus.[96] At least one immuno-inhibiting substance from *C. albicans* itself is known,[97] and T-lymphocytes, especially helper T-cells, continue to be implicated in the role of protecting the body from the growth of *Candida albicans*.[98, 99]

An ongoing study of CFS patients by the National Institute of Allergy and Infectious Diseases (NIAID) found a significant difference in the size of the population of circulating T-cells called CD4+T-lymphocytes, or helper T-cells, compared to that of normal people. A close examination found the missing T-cells had become activated, left the bloodstream, and embedded themselves in tissues. As to what could have caused this, NIAID scientists speculate that neurohormonal or neuropsychiatric factors may be involved, or even exposure to some kind of infectious agent. They noted that the change in location of these T-cells might help to explain some common CFS symptoms, such as joint and muscle pains and lymph node tenderness, for once inside of tissues the helper T-cell releases chemical messengers that are known to cause pain and mild inflammation. Inflammatory bowel disease, attended by intestinal pains, is caused by the same sort of T-cell abnormality.[100, 101]

An abnormally reduced immunologic responsiveness in lymphocytes from CFS patients confirms what many private researchers have been observing all along: this disease is an immune dysfunction syndrome. Curiously enough, the NIAID study found the same immunologic problem in people with debilitating fatigue who didn't have enough symptoms to fully qualify as CFS patients.[102] With the vast majority of EI, yeast syndrome, and CFS patients all suffering from fatigue, diarrhea, and constipation, a similar or the same T-cell problem becomes all the more likely. It follows that activating the immune system may offer a means of "distracting" the otherwise occupied helper T-cells from the tissues they irritate. But even a supposed immunostimulating action was not why people in the United States first decided to try pau d'arco bark against yeast syndrome.

What prompted this application represents another chapter in the history of medical paradoxes. It can be traced to the curious observations of Dr. Octaviano Gaiarsa,[103] a pharmacist at the Hospital of Santo André in Brazil. As reported in O'Cruzeiro, Dr. Gaiarsa stated that unlike any other type of plant, spores, "from which mushrooms originate," would not grow on pau d'arco trees and that repeated efforts to induce their growth proved fruitless, "a fact that suggests its unusual resistance."[104] This prompted an herbalist returning from Brazil to tell Gail Nielsen and others that the bark might be useful against fungal problems.[105]

Although it was not reported in the media, Dr. Gaiarsa *had* collected "mushroom samples which adhered to the rough bark" and managed to cultivate them.[106] Were it also known that Huastec Mayans of Mexico gather an edible fungus from the trunks of fallen pau d'arco,[107] I doubt that use of the bark against fungal infections would have been suggested. Examining an assortment of fresh, unprocessed pau d'arco barks, I found mold and fungi on every sample, whether inner or outer bark. Wondering if these might affect the tea, I wrote to Dr. Gaiarsa. He replied, "The mushrooms do not in any way modify the extracts or the teas because they are destroyed by the heat and by the chemical reagents."[108] By "reagents" he refers to alcohol in the "extract" preparations. But mold grows on the liquid tea if it's not refrigerated, and since even extracts will eventually become moldy (sour), they too must be refrigerated once opened.

The paradox doesn't stop there. Repeated tests have shown that pau d'arco teas and extracts are not active against *Candida*. More than a dozen samples failed to show any activity against *Candida albicans* in cultures of the fungus, with or without nystatin.[109, 110] These tests (with unprocessed botanical samples and with commercial barks purchased in the United States) were performed using every kind of method of preparation suggested, and still there was no activity.[111] It should be noted that the tests were conducted in petri dishes, which is a far cry from a living body. As such, they don't tell us that the bark is necessarily *useless* against *Candida*, but they do tell us that the mechanism of the bark against *Candida* in a living system remains to be elucidated. The bark may be active against the fungus only once *inside* a living system, or in what is known as a "host-mediated" action. This is typical of herbal medicines that stimulate cells of the immune system. In turn, those cells take action against various agents of disease: tumor cells, viruses, bacteria, and pathogenic fungi.

The fact that pau d'arco stimulates immune cells known as macrophages may be significant to its use against *Candida*:[112, 113] the macrophage performs the greatest workload in conferring resistance to *Candida*, with participation from T-cells and antibody-producing B-cells,[114] and macrophage-stimulating immunomodulators have shown the most promise in experiments to protect the body against systemic *C. albicans* infection.[115] But that isn't to say another action of the bark couldn't be at work. Today, studies are being planned in the United States to find the activities of pau d'arco in people, the deciding frontier.[116] The answers to questions held far too long are eagerly anticipated.

Both *The Yeast Syndrome* (Bantam Books, 1986) by John Parks Trowbridge, M.D., and *The Yeast Connection* (Professional Books, 1983) by William G. Crook, M.D., include a number of other natural products and products containing pau d'arco that people have found useful. There are numerous botanical formulas containing the bark. In 1988 I found seven herbal formulas with pau d'arco. Today there are probably a dozen or more in the United States alone.[117]

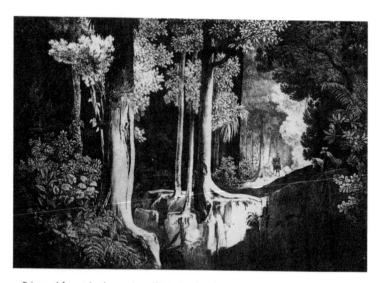

Primeval forest in the region of São Paulo of 1840–1906. From Carlos F. P. De Martius and Augustus G. Eichler, *Flora Brasiliensis, 1840–1906,* vol. 1, part 1 (Weinheim, Germany: Verlag von J. Cramer, 1965), reprint.

THREE

FOREST PHARMACY

In this episode we'll journey through the tropical Americas to learn the different ways pau d'arco trees are presently used by those who have known them as remedies the longest, the Indians. While it is true that the bark has been found to stimulate the immune system, a subject taken up later on, it will become obvious that this is not pau d'arco's only action. Bear in mind that the bark remains, as is the case for so many South American herbs, scarcely studied. Yet there is hope, for the most promising clues to pau d'arco's medicinal secrets are evident in folk medicine.

PAU D'ARCO

Pau d'arco comprises a group of trees known to botanists by the Latin names *Tabebuia* (tab-eb-ū-ee-ah) and *Tecoma*. Pau d'arco or lapacho trees were generally described by the tropical forester Samuel J. Record:[1, 2]

> This group is represented in all parts of continental tropical America and some of the Lesser Antilles. Many closely related species have been described, but from the standpoint of their woods the number could be greatly reduced. All are trees, usually of medium to large size with well-formed trunks . . . the flowers are mostly yellow, sometimes pink, red, or violet; the fruit is a long woody capsule with winged seeds. The timber is noted for its great strength and durability. The vessels contain an abundance of yellow powder (lapachol compound) which looks like sulpher [sic] but in the presence of alkaline solutions turns deep red.[3]

Pau d'arco are well known in Brazil, where they often decorate streets and boulevards. Brazilians call them *ipés* (ee-pays), *pau-d'arco*, or *ipé-roxo* (eepay-rosho) to denote the purple-flowered varieties, the kind Professor Accorsi decided were the "more efficient" against leukemia.[4] But purple pau d'arco aren't always purple. Although *roxo* proper means "purple" in Portuguese,[5] the language of Brazil, the people use the term rather loosely to include pink-, red-, magenta-, and violet-flowered varieties.[6]

The wood was widely used by native archers to make bows,[7] an application preserved in the name *pau d'arco*, which translates "bow stick."[8] At one time, there was a group of the Kayapo Indian tribe in Brazil called the Pau d'Arco, but contact with white missionaries proved to be their downfall: their number rapidly fell from 1,500 to a few people when epidemics to which they had no immunity ravaged their communities.[9] Meteors, thunder, and rainbows held great meaning for the Pau d'Arco, and their shamans were known as "Wonderworkers who commune with snakes, jaguars, and other beings and exert great influence." By not taking their "powers" from departed souls, they were distinguished from the shamans of many other tribes.[10] In the state of Piauí in northern Brazil, Lake Pau d'Arco now bears the name of this extinct tribe.

Pau d'arco are timber trees, providing a high-quality wood.[11] They grow to 150 feet with trunks to six feet in diameter.[12] According to the world authority on the botany of *Tabebuia*, the late Alwyn H. Gentry (1945–93), curator of the Missouri Botanical Garden in St. Louis, "*Tabebuia* have perhaps the hardest, heaviest, most durable wood of any neotropical tree."[13] The guayacan (*Tabebuia guayacan*), for example, has a characteristically high resistance to termites,[14] and the heartwood is also highly resistant to decay by fungi.[15] Their wood is so durable that beams left exposed for nearly three centuries were discovered "perfectly sound."[16] Giving a handsome finish, the woods of pau d'arco have been used in everything from the construction of boats to farm tools[17] and the paneling of many Latin American banks, finer homes, and stores.[18]

The trees themselves are adored, especially in bloom. During a visit to Argentina after his presidency, Theodore Roosevelt was at once so enraptured by the extraordinary beauty of the pau d'arco blooming along the streets of Buenos Aires that he immediately requested seeds to grow his own in the United States.[19] So esteemed are they by tropical American countries, many adopted pau d'arco as a national symbol. Brazil has the striking yellow-flowered *Tabebuia serratifolia*, and El Salvador the showy pink to purple-flowered *T. rosea*. Other countries include Ecuador (*T. chrysantha*), Paraguay (*T. heptaphylla*), and Venezuela (*T. billbergi*),[20] while for both the Virgin Islands and the Bahamas a closely related tree or shrub known as yellow bells (*Tecoma stans*) holds the title of national flower.[21, 22] The same plant is the main anti-diabetic remedy of Mexican folk medicine.[23, 24] Many cures are reported from a tea made of the flowers and leaves or bark.[25, 26]

In Argentina, *T. impetiginosa* loses all its leaves during May or early June and from then to August it blooms with great clusters of violet-pink flowers.[27] But the majority of pau d'arco are evergreens: regardless of the time of year, they're rarely bare. Even those that lose their leaves at once

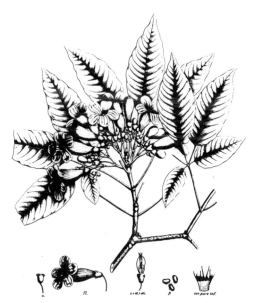

Tabebuia impetiginosa. From Carlos F. P. De Martius
and Augustus G. Eichler, *Flora Brasiliensis, 1896–1897,* vol 8, part 2
(Weinheim, Germany: Verlag von J. Cramer, 1967), reprint.

become a bouquet of flowers.[28] Gentry explains that they occur more abundantly in tropical climes and bloom, opening "all or almost all their flowers on the same day . . . and are completely covered with a profusion of blossoms which typically last only a few days." Otherwise, they "flower in coordinated bursts scattered throughout the year."[29]

HARVEST

The inner bark, or cortex, of a tree has a primary function of storing food and water and eventually of becoming outer bark as the tree grows older. The cortex of pau d'arco ranges in color from a deep reddish brown or simple brown to a sandy pink, sometimes with sections of a straw-like color and of a charcoal gray, although it seems not in all species. General appearance will vary in accord with the wood and with age, species, and ecological factors peculiar to the region of harvest. One characteristic I have noticed between the layers of inner bark is calcium oxalate in the form of prismatic crystals, which in some samples I examined from Brazil were fairly large—larger than the ones commonly found on the underside of spinach leaves.

The inner barks of yellow-flowered pau d'arco show a straw-like color throughout, and, although it may be rare, I found a distinctly purple coloration in a small section of inner bark from the "purple" pau d'arco of northeast Argentina (*Tabebuia ipe* [Mart.] Standley = *T. heptaphylla* [Vellozo] Toledo). Coincidentally or not, the wood of this tree is known to produce a dye with a purplish color.[30] In Brazil, the barks of various pau d'arco still find use as a dye source,[31] usually giving cloth a yellow coloration.

The native preference for the inner bark over the outer bark appears to be widespread. Thousands of miles away, on the northwest coast of Canada, the Salish Indians hold the belief that the true medicine of a tree is found in the cortex, "the softer, moister, lighter coloured inner portion of the bark." Canadian ethnobotanist Nancy J. Turner explains that the Indians believe that to obtain medicinal barks of "maximum effectiveness," one should harvest early in the morning before one has eaten. It is a common practice for the bark to be taken from the trunk side that first receives the morning rays of the sun. The Salishan believe that the side receiving the most sun "heals over [re-grows bark] more quickly." Turner writes that added to this piece of conservation, the Indians take only "a small strip" of bark from a tree, thereby shortening the time needed by the tree to heal. Two Salish herbalists told her that the sores or other disease of the patient "will heal just as the tree itself heals."[32]

A similar procedure for removing the bark of pau d'arco was left by Teodoro Meyer. From instructions provided by his son, the method he practiced in Argentina, which allowed the bark to grow back and spared the tree, consisted of removing only as much as a third of the bark surface of the tree.[33]

PURPLE PAU D'ARCO

The main species of purple pau d'arco used medicinally in Brazil are kindly designated for me by Professor Valter Accorsi as *Tabebuia avellanedae*, *T. heptaphylla*, and *T. roseo-alba*. The one used more than any other is *Tabebuia avellanedae* (avay-an-eday),[34] which is now correctly known as *Tabebuia impetiginosa*.[35] Even the name *impetiginosa* refers to a medicinal use of the tree, specifically against impetigo,[36] a staph or strep infection of the skin also called impetigo contagiosa. Medically, *avellanedae* is meaningless. It is simply a suburb in the south of Buenos Aires where the tree was first identified in Argentina,[37] a place named in honor of General Nicolas Avellanedae (1836–85), one of Argentina's more benevolent presidents.[38]

It is significant to find native peoples hundreds and even thousands of miles apart using pau d'arco trees for the same or very similar conditions. Armed with the knowledge of what various doctors in Brazil observed, as well as North American accounts, we can now look for corroboration from Indian uses and find those of their applications with more assured effect.

ROBLE COLORADO

One of the most eye-filling examples is the "roble colorado" (*Tabebuia rosea* [Bertol.] A. P. Candolle). This tree makes its homeland from northern Venezuela to coastal Ecuador and southern Mexico. *Roble* is the Spanish name for oak, and the furrowed dark gray of the outer bark along with the heavy brown wood certainly fits the namesake.[39] This pau d'arco usually has yellow-throated flowers, "pale pink or red-purple."[40]

Costa Ricans take a decoction (boiled or simmered preparation) of the bark for the treatment of colds, headaches, fever, and constipation. The flowers, leaves, and roots provide a decoction that they drink for the treatment of snakebite. They also apply this externally.[41] In Panama, the bark is used as a treatment for boils, dysentery, pharyngitis, and wounds and as a fungicide. In Guatemala, a decoction of the bark is regularly given to dogs as a protection against rabies. Mexicans make a decoction of the bark along with the leaves to reduce temperature in fevers,[42] and while the bark is used to treat pain,[43] a root decoction is employed to remedy anemia.[44]

In South America, Colombians use the bark infusion (steeped preparation) or decoction as a gargle for diseases of the throat, and the tea is also taken to treat fevers.[45] The bark contains a high amount of tannin and has demonstrated stimulation of the central nervous system as well as antibiotic activity against a type of fungi that attacks the nails, hair, and skin (*Trichophyton mentagrophytes*), but it was inactive against *Candida albicans*.[46]

The tannin content of the bark is an important factor in applications against throat diseases and external sores and wounds. Tannic acid has been used as an "astringent for the mucus membrane of the mouth and throat," and it was once a common treatment for diarrhea.[47]

Among the tannins in pau d'arco are condensed tannins or "catechins",[48] which are also known as a type of flavonol. Colorless and water soluble,[49] catechin is an astringent principle (causing contraction of tissues) primarily found in flowering woody plants.[50] Catechins appear to act as protectants in bark and wood against the ravages of normal decay and infections.[51] They are abundant in the leaves of the common willow (*Salix caprea*), the skins of many fruits and berries,[52] tea (green and black), red wine, and hawthorn berries.[53] The seeds of mature grapes are a major source of catechins for the cosmetic and pharmaceutical industry,[54] and you can find grape seed oil in various body lotions and phyto-cosmetics. Another rich source is the root of rhatany (*Krameria triadra* Ruiz and Pav.), a South American shrub found in Bolivia, Brazil, Colombia, and Peru that produces a product used to tan leathers. This plant is traditionally used for varicose ulcers, wounds, and inflammations,[55] and the oil extracted from the root has an ultraviolet (UV) filtering action comparable to some of the most potent synthetic UV filters available.[56]

The biological activity of catechins has been described as "remarkably high."[57] They will even show activity in minute amounts.[58, 59] At inhibiting the peroxidation of lipids (fats) in liver cells, catechin tannin was five times as potent as vitamin E. Lipid peroxides cause injuries to the blood vessels (arteriosclerosis), kidneys, and liver.[60] As a drug (cianidanol), catechin has been applied in Europe to treat hepatitis.[61]

In a comparative study with several other bioflavonoids (rutin, hesperidin, and esculin) topically applied to the skin, catechins were found "the most active." In decreasing abnormal bleeding, capillary fragility (of small blood vessels), and symptoms of shock, catechins remained active even when partly decomposed.[62] In high amounts, catechins[63] and some other types of tannins have shown antitumor,[64–66] antimutagenic,[67] cholesterol-lowering,[68] antibacterial,[69] iron chelating,[70] blood-flow increasing,[71] and still other potentially therapeutic actions.[72–74]

Injected into the stomach region (peritoneum) of rodents, a water extract of the bark of a yellow pau d'arco, the paratodu or caraiba of Brazil[75] (*Tabebuia aurea*)[76] showed definite antitumor activity. Two condensed tannins appear to have been largely responsible. These were determined as peonidin and an unidentified, closely related compound.[77] Condensed tannins have also been isolated from the barks of pink-flowered pau d'arco[78, 79] along with peonidin compounds from the flowers,[80, 81] but their activities remain to be studied. More technically known as an anthocyanidin, peonidin is one of the major pigments in the skins of the purple sweet potato (*Ipomoea batatas*). Taking its name from peony plants (*Paeonia* sp.), peonidin is widely distributed in the plant kingdom as a pigment providing a violet-blue to reddish purple tone to many flowers. For this reason peonidin may be valuable as a food dye.[82]

Another cofactor to consider in topical applications is that of calcium oxalate, which is clearly visible and fairly abundant in the bark cortex of pau d'arco trees as tiny, shiny white crystals.[83] One medical historian has suggested that calcium oxalate in plants used to treat cancer in antiquity provided a cleansing action upon external sores.[84]

MEDICINE OF THE HUASTEC MAYANS

The roble colorado (*Tabebuia rosea*) grows in, among other locations, northern Veracruz and southeast San Luis Potosí in Mexico. There, ethnobotanist Janis B. Alcorn studied firsthand the present-day uses of plant medicines by Mayan-speaking Huastecs, an Indian people living today as peasants. Her many fascinating observations include their application of this pau d'arco in the form of a bark decoction "used as a douche" to treat cancer of the uterus or vagina. Although they recognize a white-flowered variety, only the bark from pink-flowered pau d'arco is regarded useful.[85, 86]

The bark decoction is applied as a wash on wounds and sores and is drunk to treat malaise, ulcers, and cancer.[87–89] The common name is *k'uul*, and a fungus the Indians call *tsikinte*, found on the trunks of fallen stands, is collected for food.[90] In their treatment of sores, Alcorn noticed that besides making use of the leaves, they shave the bark and toast it before applying it directly to the area affected. This is performed after washing the sore with a leaf tea from *tsul te'* (*Cecropia obtusifolia*).[91] At this we are reminded of how the bark of the tepeschuite (*Mimosa tenuiflora*) was also treated with fire before being applied topically to treat burns. The Mexican practice of subjecting herbal material to fire may have no pharmacologic advantage. But to the healer and the patient, the "energy" imparted to the medicine affects ancient traditional beliefs.[92]

When they feel "generally" sick, the Huastec Mayan prepare a pau d'arco bath. They boil the bark along with four other plants: a shrub used for skin disease (*Cestrum dumentorum* Schlecht.); a plant used for "kidney trouble" and "inner fever" (*Paramentiera edulis* DC.); a tree bark (*Piscidia piscipula* [L.] Sarg.) known as a "tonic," which is also used to treat vertigo and dysentery; and the scented *Cedrela odorata* tree, which is used for chills, edema (the bark), cold feet, and malaise (the leaves).[93]

Alcorn found that the bark was also prescribed for diseases classified as *jaluk'laab*, which she explains might be called "magical diseases." The term translates as "soul exchange," but she says there is no doubt that persons so diagnosed are ill. Alcorn explains that these are conditions diagnosed in patients "who are more seriously ill but who exhibit a wide range of symptoms."[94] Otherwise, the patient is "very ill" or "sleepy." For the treatment of jaluk'laab, they boil the bark in water with the addition of *aguardiente* (cane liquor) and two other plants (*Cedrela odorata* L. and *Trichilia havanensis* Jacq., a small tree). The decoction is kept covered, cooled until warm, and then the patient is bathed with it. Aspirin or "Manzaniya tea" (chamomile) is taken, and the patient is covered while a fever with sweating occurs. The patient musn't go outdoors or get up for seventy-two hours and then must adhere to a "special diet" for another eight days before returning to a normal diet. Coffee and greasy foods are prohibited. Should the fever persist past twenty-four hours, the patient drinks a tea made from the bark of a tree called *tsitsiy* (*Chlorophora tinctoria* [L.] Gaud).[95]

The Huastecs' herbal formulas are prepared daily using fresh plant materials. They thoroughly crush the material and then make their teas with but a small amount of water. Remedies taken internally are first tested with three doses a day over three days, at which point a judgement is made of efficacy.[96] A cup or so is taken before sleep and once before each meal. Dosage is determined by the age, sex, and size of the patient, and the common practice is to leave the plant parts used steeping in the tea.[97]

However *natural* their lifestyle, these people have a cancer rate approximately that in the United States, and arthritis, allergies, fungal infections, and tuberculosis are very common year round.[98] Perhaps in learning why we may turn up answers to the prevalence of the same diseases here.

Before moving on, the matter of safety should concern anyone wishing to make use of these Mayan remedies, at least until more is known.

Toward that end, a few facts about the use of these plants in folk medicine will be useful.

Tsul te' (*Cecropia obtusifolia*) provides a leaf tea used to wash sores.[99] Some Indians have made a decoction of the young leaves of this tree to treat liver ailments.[100] A single leaf of "kooch-le" is boiled in a liter of water to provide a treatment for asthma, edema, obesity, kidney problems, and diabetes. The decoction is used as a tonic in Yucatan and is also applied to relieve fever, promote sweating and menstruation, and hasten child delivery. Herbalists in Guatemala use the decoction for the relief of respiratory "allergy." The leaves contain a cardiotonic substance (ambain) and have central nervous system calming, diuretic, and antiatherogenic activity. The sap from the trunk is caustic enough to remove warts, a use common in Mexico.[101] In the Peruvian Amazon, species of *Cecropia* are known for their resin. Various species are applied as antiseptics, and the juice is applied on wounds to stop bleeding and is used to treat abscesses.[102]

The plants used with pau d'arco by the Huastec Mayans in baths when feeling "generally" sick clearly have diverse actions and must be approached with caution.[103] For example, some *Cestrum* species are used for everything from fish poisons to insecticides, cancer treatments, diarrhea, fevers, dental abscesses, and arthritis.[104] At least one species is considered by the Indians of Colombia as being "virulently toxic,"[105] and ranchers in El Salvador regard the same species used by the Huastec Mayans as toxic to their cattle. Mexicans and Guatemalans decoct the new shoots and leaves of this ill-smelling shrub for application on "skin diseases."[106]

The candle tree (*Paramentiera edulis*) is a member of the same family pau d'arco belongs to (Bignoniaceae), and the Huastec Mayans are by no means the only ones to find this small tree useful. In the Peruvian Amazon the fruits are eaten as a diuretic, to cool the body, and as a food.[107] The bark has been applied to treat typhoid fever, and both the fruit and the leaves are used in Mexican folk medicine to treat edema. The Mexicans use a hot beverage of the boiled fruits for kidney stones and any urinary problems. Both the leaf decoction and the juice are used for indigestion, and the juice is put into the ears to treat deafness or inflammation. The root tea or decoction is regarded as effective for snakebite and diabetes.[108]

More than one bath ingredient used by the Huastec Mayans with pau d'arco may have been added with relaxing the patient in mind. One example is *Piscidia piscipula*. As noted earlier, the bark of this tree is regarded as a "tonic" and is used to treat vertigo and dysentery.[109] The roots and powdered bark of *Piscidia* were once used by the Carib Indians to stupify fish. A compound named piscidin was found as the main sleep-inducing factor, an action reflected in the common name — fishfuddle tree.[110] The bark of the barbasco smells similar to opium, and the tree contain several toxins. On the Yucatan peninsula, the bark extract is used in drops for a sedative and sweat-promoting effect. The dried root has been used to relieve the pain of aching teeth, and various preparations derived from the root or dried bark have been utilized in pharmaceutical products to "successfully" treat everything from chronic bronchitis to whooping cough, neuralgia, headaches, insomnia, hysteria, chronic alcoholism, and pain from bone fractures, surgery, and pregnancy.[111] Indeed, opium has had at least as many different uses but owing to toxic components isn't the best of medicines, either. I suspect topical applications are the safest way to use this plant.

In the Caribbean, the root of the West Indian cedar (*Cedrela odorata*) is taken to treat fevers.[112] In the Peruvian Amazon, the same tree is regarded as an emetic and is used to treat gangrene.[113] This plant, along with *Tabebuia rosea* and *Trichilia havanensis*, is the one used as a bath by Huastec Mayan herbalists for patients with jaluk'laab, a so-called magical disease.[114] A bark tea of the acajou tree (*Cedrela odorata* L.) is drunk to relieve chronic headaches accompanying menstrual periods and to stimulate the appetite. In Mexico, the tea is used for diarrhea, dyspepsia, indigestion, hemorrhages, vomiting, and bronchitis. The bark powder is utilized for "bathing" ulcers and wounds, and the leaf tea is used in Yucatan to treat pyorrhea and toothache. In Jamaica the twigs and leaves are added to baths to give relief from "pains" and fever.[115]

Trichilia species are noted more for their wood than for medicinal purposes.[116] The trees are well known in Africa, where the seeds of the Natal mahogany (*T. emetica* Vahl) provide a hair and body oil also used for cooking and in soaps. The oil is ingested to treat rheumatism and applied externally on cuts and bone fractures. The bark tea is used to induce vomiting, and the leaf tea is taken for coughs and applied as a lotion for bruises.[117] Ethnobotanist Julia F. Morton lists folk uses of this tree in the tropical Americas for similar purposes. Guatemalans add the leaf decoction to hot baths for the relief of rheumatism, and they use the bark decoction to remedy malaria. In Costa Rica a decoction of the bark is used for bladder ailments, and the leaf decoction is taken to remedy kidney stones, inflammation of the urinary tract, and hematuria (bloody urine). The same preparation is used externally to treat skin diseases.[118]

Alcorn notes that the persistence of fever in the patient with jaluk'laab is treated with a bark tea of *Cholorphora tinctoria*.[119] The same plant is known in the Peruvian Amazon as incira, an astringent, diuretic, purgative, analgesic, yellow dye source, antisyphilitic, antirheumatic, and tonic with edible fruit.[120] In Panama[121] and in Peru, the tree sap is applied directly to remove rotten teeth without pain or bleeding.[122]

From the foregoing brief introductions, it should be clear that there is a need for much more research before these plants can be utilized with safety as herbal medicines. Their topical or "transdermal" application in herbal baths merits investigation, both because this method of treatment is widespread among Indians of the Americas and has scarcely been studied, and because the immune system, of which the skin is the largest component organ, is modulated by T-cells (T-lymphpocytes) that reside in and maintain the health of our skin.[123–125] It is also known that herbs extracted with water are rich in low-molecular-weight compounds with low melting points, and these are the properties of drugs that are the most readily absorbed transdermally.[126,127]

CARIBBEAN CONCOCTIONS

The pink trumpet (*Tabebuia bahamensis* [Northrop] Britton),[128,129] also called big man, above all, five finger, and a host of other names,[130,131] is famous on Andros Island in the Bahamas as a principal ingredient of an herbal aphrodisiac that is also taken whenever one feels weak. Mainly used by men, the tree is regarded in Jamaica and Trinidad for the same purpose.[132] Low libido being a common symptom in depression, this pau d'arco is currently listed by Brazilian pharmacologists as a plant with "potential antidepressant activity": a candidate for studies to uncover new sources of antidepressant drugs.[133] Its flowers are "pale magenta" and occasionally white.[134] Bahamians boil the leaves for a remedy commonly applied in headache, gonorrhea, and toothache, and a bark decoction or an "infusion" (prepared by steeping the plant part like ordinary tea) is taken as a tonic for strength. A decoction of the leaves is used as a fish poisoning antidote in Curaçao, and both the bark and leaves are ingredients of herbal aphrodisiacs. Energizing tonics are often prepared with the leaves and bark of this pau d'arco combined with the leaves and/or bark[135] of the strong back tree (*Bourreiria ovata* Miers), an evergreen with ivory-white flowers.[136]

Not far away, in St. Kitts, the bark and leaves of another purple pau d'arco, the shrubby *T. pallida* (Lindley) Miers, are boiled to prepare a "cure" for the common cold.[137]

YELLOW PAU D'ARCO

After one of the stories in *O'Cruzeiro* stated that though the purple pau d'arco is more efficient, both the purple and the yellow are medicinal, the bark of the pau d'arco amarelo, a yellow-flowered tree (*Tabebuia serratifolia* [Vahl] Nichols.),[138] was also commercialized and torn from trunks across Brazil[139, 140]—regardless of its status as the country's national symbol. (In the city of Campinas it didn't seem to matter what the species was: every pau d'arco in the vicinity was stripped until the trunks were completely bare.[141])

Although Professor Accorsi could have compared any species of pau d'arco, after more than twenty years' experience with these trees, he insists the *amarélo* (yellow) are simply "no good."[142] Sources in Brazil affirm his stand, adding that in the botanical gardens one will often find the *amarélos* left untouched, whereas the *roxo* (purple) will be missing large sections of bark, literally ripped off by the public.[143] It remains the case, however, that in Brazil and other parts of the tropical Americas there are *amarélos* that the natives uphold as medicines.

A survey of herb use in the regional area around the capital city of Brasilia in 1981 found the inner bark of both a purple and a yellow species (*T. aurea*) used as diuretics and as remedies for ulcers.[144] The bark tea (infusion) of the yellow-flowered *jadujedi* (*Tabebuia chrysantha* [Jacq.] Nichols.) is used by the Yanomani Indians of Venezuela "to cure stomachache,"[145] and the bark of the *apamate* (*T. insignis* [Miq.] Sandu var. *insignis*), a white-flowered pau d'arco,[146] is used by the Warao Indians of eastern Venezuela to treat bloody dysentery, diarrhea, and scorpion stings.[147] The bark tea made from a different variety of the same tree (*T. insignis* var. *monophylla* Sandwith) in central and eastern Colombia is locally regarded as "excellent" for treating stomach ulcers. In the same region of northwest Amazonia, women of the Taiwanos Indian tribe add the dried yellow flowers of "tahuarí" (*T. obscura* [Bur. and K. Schum.] Sandwith) to their food to remedy irregular menstruation, and the Boras Indians of Peru believe the bark of this tree is "antirheumatic." Finally, the Tikuna Indians of the northwest Amazon learned to use the bark decoction of the golden yellow–flowered *hua-ri* (*T. ochracea* ssp. *neochrysanthea* [A. Gentry]) for chronic anemia, malaria, and ulcer pains by taking only an "eighth of a cup" three times daily.[148] This tree has yellow flowers with fine red lines in the throat and occurs in dry forests from El Salvador to northwest Venezuela.[149]

American herbal authority Dr. James A. Duke has records showing the same yellow pau d'arco (*T. serratifolia*) that was mentioned in *O'Cruzeiro* being "used traditionally for cancer in Colombia."[150] According to the *Flora Medicinal de Colombia*, the bark of that tree, called *palo de arco*, "is employed as an anticarcinogen in infusion [tea] or decoction [boiled or simmered]."[151] From his many expeditions in the Amazon, the report of famous Harvard ethnobotanist Wade Davis, whose real-life investigation of a voodoo formula inspired the Hollywood movie *Serpent and the Rainbow*, is much the same:

> Throughout the Amazon, the bark of *T. serratifolia* is taken as a decoction or infusion to cure cancer. It is believed to be so effective that it is regularly prescribed by both folk and western doctors.[152]

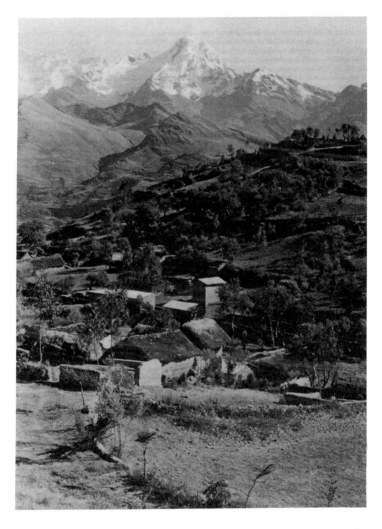

A village of the Kallawayas at the foothills of the Bolivian Andes. Courtesy of Joseph W. Bastien. From *Healers of the Andes* by Joseph W. Bastien (Salt Lake City: University of Utah Press, 1987), 8.

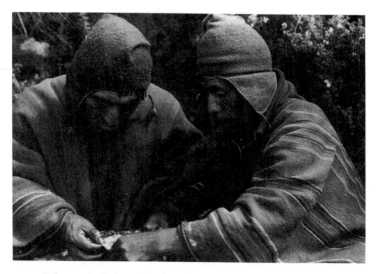

Kallawaya herbalist and patient discerning a diagnosis. Courtesy of
Joseph W. Bastien. From *Drum and Stethoscope* by Joseph W. Bastien
(Salt Lake City: University of Utah Press, 1992), 79.

MEDICINE OF THE KALLAWAYA

The *Quollhuaya* ("Kallawaya") herbalists of the Bolivian Andes are noted
as "the most renowned" in all of South America.[153, 154] Their name means
"man who travels with medicine on his shoulders."[155] Their practice goes
back over ten centuries, and today at least 1,000 plants make up their
prescriptions. With so long a tradition and great acclaim, they are hon-
ored by the peoples of the Andes as *Qolla Kapachayuh*—Lords of the
Medicine Bag.[156]

The American authority on these people is Dr. Joseph W. Bastien, a
sociologist at the University of Texas at Arlington. Living among them, he
cataloged hundreds of plant medicines.[157] He found that like many South
American folk healers today, they do not object to modern medicines
and will advise their patients to obtain surgery, antibiotics, vitamins, and
other contemporary treatments, although often combined with herbs. A

patient with a venereal disease, for example, would be given a prescription for penicillin along with certain herbs.[158] Highly resourceful, they had previously made use of molds.[159] Archaeologists uncovered their distant past to find evidence of brain surgery and the application of plants for anesthesia, achievements showing a history rich in the pursuit of medical command.[160]

Dr. Bastien recounts that by the early 1900s, Kallawaya medicine had achieved international fame.[161] One of the more critical events was the Eighth World Exposition in Paris in 1889, where an inventory of Kallawaya plant medicines was received by the European community from two doctors engaged in cataloging the Kallawaya pharmacopeia. It was published by the Geographical Society of La Paz in 1904. Shaping the reputation of the Kallawaya abroad, "cures" were naturally the more deciding event. Bastien relates the case of a crippled girl who had four operations on her hip by German physicians, apparently to no benefit. Her cure in only one week by a Kallawaya who employed medicinal plants and compresses served to legendize Andean medicine,[162] and the mystique persists to this day.

During construction of the Panama Canal, Kallawaya herbalists were sent to treat canal workers plagued with yellow fever. Following their success in curing the workers with tree bark (*Cinchona micrantha*, or "Peruvian bark," the source of quinine), the hopeful who had been given up as incurable began arriving from all over South America and as far away as Europe. For a time, the world believed these Lords of the Medicine Bag could cure anything. But as Dr. Bastien explains, their successful image was bolstered by the fact that they refused to treat a patient who was unlikely to survive, or when they could discern that their medicine would not suffice.[163]

Later, as pharmacists and physicians began to increase in Bolivia, Kallawaya medicine came under attack.[164] A smear campaign painted its practitioners as backward or, worse, as "witch doctors," which the people associated with evil. Portrayed as defiants standing in the way of "scientific medicine," their practice was prohibited. For years there were arrests and short imprisonments.[165] But with public recognition from the Boliv-

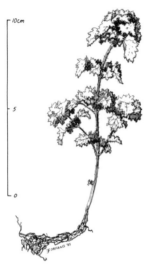

Ortega blanca is one of the
ingredients of a Kallawaya recipe
using pau d'arco. It is a species of nettle
(*Urtica flabellata* H.B.K.) found in the Bolivian
Andes. Courtesy of Joseph W. Bastien. From
Healers of the Andes by Joseph W. Bastien
(Salt Lake City: University of Utah Press, 1987),
65. Drawing by Eleanor Forfang Stauffer.

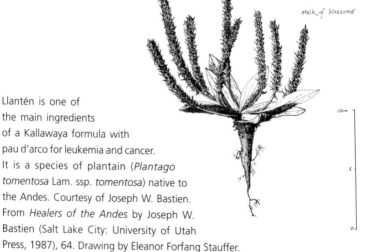

Llantén is one of
the main ingredients
of a Kallawaya formula with
pau d'arco for leukemia and cancer.
It is a species of plantain (*Plantago
tomentosa* Lam. ssp. *tomentosa*) native to
the Andes. Courtesy of Joseph W. Bastien.
From *Healers of the Andes* by Joseph W.
Bastien (Salt Lake City: University of Utah
Press, 1987), 64. Drawing by Eleanor Forfang Stauffer.

ian president, a major turning point for the Kallawaya occurred in 1956, and now their tradition is growing.[166]

Andeans are a people filled with superstition, and choice of diagnostic methods can vary from one herbalist to the next. Like healers in many parts of South America, the Kallawayas diagnose by divination. At some point, however, their treatments are based on the physiological effects of herbs handed down for centuries.[167] The number of plants they use that offer "effective cures" has been estimated at 25 to 30 percent of over 1,000 different herbs.[168] According to Bastien, "Herbalists claim that pharmaceutical companies have utilized more than 50 species from the [Kallawaya] pharmacopeia for use in manufacturing drugs."[169] For this they have yet to receive so much as a single royalty in remuneration.[170]

TAJIBO

To obtain the bark of a pau d'arco they call *tajibo* (taheebo),[171] which is also the name of a tribe of the Guarani Indians, Bolivian Kallawaya descend from their residence over 9,000 feet above sea level and travel to Santa Cruz at the foothills of the Andes.[172] Samples at this time have not been identified according to species[173] (possibly *T. impetiginosa*, *T. rosea-alba*, or *T. serratifolia*),[174] but Dr. Bastien has learned their use. By Kallawaya understanding, tajibo is a medicine that purifies the blood and whose principal use is as a treatment for leukemia. Often, they mix the bark with the leaves of *ortega blanca*,[175] a kind of nettle (*Urtica flabellata*) native to the Andes that they apply to fractures and wounds in the form of a poultice. As a tea for patients with tuberculosis,[176] the flowers are boiled along with red nettle flowers (*ortega colorado*, *Cajophora* sp.), a glass to be taken three times daily. The same formula is applied to treat uterine and ovarian irritations.[177]

Against leukemia and cancer, one Andean recipe calls for five grams each of white nettle leaves (*ortega blanca*, *Urtica flabellata* H.B.K), plantago leaves (*llantén*, *Plantago tomentosa* Lam. ssp. *tomentosa*), and the bark of tajibo. The mixture is boiled for a full fifteen minutes in water (one liter) and allowed to cool before drinking; half a "glass" to be taken three times daily.[178, 179] In the treatment of malaria and fevers, including typhoid and yellow fever, the remedy is prepared as above using ten grams of each herb boiled in half the amount of water.[180]

Species of nettle and plantago are found in many parts of the world and systems of herbal medicine. Stinging nettle root (*Urtica dioica*) has shown beneficial effects against prostate cancer in elderly patients,[181] and in laboratory studies an extract of the dried or fresh root has shown immunostimulating activity, as well as fever and inflammation-counteracting effects.[182] The freeze-dried extract was found to be clinically effective against the symptoms of hay fever (allergic rhinitis).[183] Stinging nettle has also shown strong inhibitory action against the viruses HIV and cytomegalovirus, a type of herpesvirus.[184] Other species of nettle are likely to have the same actions.

The roots and leaves of *Plantago major* were tested for activities ascribed in folk medicine, such as a pain-relieving action. Taken orally by guinea pigs, the herb showed definite analgesic effects.[185] In clinical studies in Europe, where the same *Plantago* is called bronchoplant, doctors found benefits in chronic bronchitis patients.[186] One study in twenty-five patients diagnosed with chronic bronchitis found 80 percent improved after twenty-five to thirty days on the herb. The treatment was well tolerated, and there were no signs of toxicity to kidneys, liver, blood, or the gastrointestinal tract.[187]

In Peru, llanten is a taken as a gargle for bronchial inflammation and sore throats. But for the Kallawayas, llanten (*Plantago tomentosa*) is primarily an herb that affects the stomach. They commonly use it to neutralize stomach acids,[188] an application also found for species of *Plantago* in Germany, where in 1990 it was one of the most prescribed single herbs for gastrointestinal problems.[189]

PRESCRIPTION IN PERU

Herbalists of Peru make use of several species of pau d'arco. The *palo santo*[190] (*Tabebuia ochracea* [Cham.] Standl. ssp. *ochracea*), a "gnarled and twisted" tree with tannish colored flowers,[191] is used in the treatment of rheumatism and syphilis as well as *soroche*, which is altitude or mountain sickness caused by hypoxia or a lack of oxygen. In the more

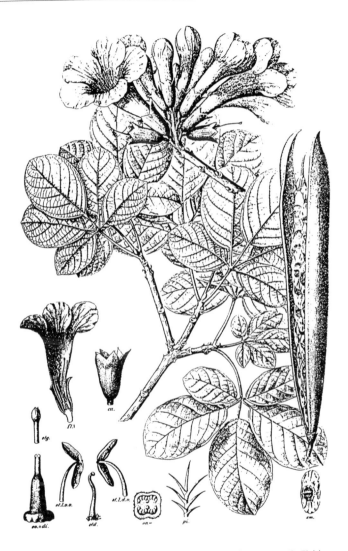

Tabebuia ochracea. From Carlos F. P. De Martius and Augustus G. Eichler, *Flora Brasiliensis, 1896–1897,* vol. 8, part 2. (Weinheim, Germany: Verlag von J. Cramer, 1967), reprint.

serious form known as high-altitude pulmonary edema, the sickness may appear as pneumonia because of fluid accumulation in the lungs. The symptoms of altitude sickness include shortness of breath, lassitude, headache, nausea, vomiting, and sleep disturbance.[192] The palo santo is also regarded by herbalists of the Peruvian Andes as a "stimulant" and as an herb to promote perspiration.[193]

In Amazonian Peru, the yellow-flowered *tauari* (*Tabebuia aurea* [Manso] Benth. and Hook. f. ex S. Moore) is used to treat syphilis.[194] The bark of the same species has been used to treat fevers and malaria and in Brazil to treat ulcers.[195] Administered orally, the bark showed moderately active against malaria in animals.[196] Another yellow species in this area, known as *palo de arco* (*Tabebuia serratifolia* [Vahl.] Nichols.), is regarded as an astringent and finds use in the treatment of cutaneous ulcers.[197]

In central Peru, an infusion of the inner bark of a pau d'arco called the *tarota* tree (*Tabebuia incana*) and that of another also called *tarota* (*T. impetiginosa*) is drunk by the Campa-Ashaninca Indians as a treatment for cancer. Against cancer, these Indians also use the *shabétoshi* (*Eupatorium macrophyllum*) and *pitirishi* (*Phyllanthus niruri*),[198] a plant that at one time was also used in India for the treatment of abdominal tumors.[199]

Various species of *Eupatorium* have shown significant antitumor activity, and many of the compounds responsible are known. One of these is eupatorin,[200] a type of bioflavonoid, and at least fifteen kinds of compounds with antitumor activity occur in six different species of *Eupatorium*. All of these belong to the group of compounds known as sesquiterpenes.[201] While other species have been examined for activity and chemical make-up,[202, 203] the shibétoshi appears to have been neglected. Cuban herbalists take a leaf decoction of this herbaceous plant to remedy colic and indigestion, while in Trinidad the crushed leaves are utilized as a suppository to treat vaginal inflammation and prolapse of the vagina. A root tea is taken to promote urination and to speed the healing process following childbirth. The roots and leaves are also combined to make a decoction for relieving fever.[204] Although some species of *Eupatorium* are utilized in folk medicine for their anti-inflammatory activity,[205] because more than one species is known to contain toxic antitumor compounds also known for causing cancer and damaging the liver,[206, 207] any *Eupatorium* should be screened for toxicity before use.

As for pitirishi, in 1993 an antitumor compound called phyllanthoside, derived from the root of a toxic relative (*Phyllanthus acuminatus* Vahl.) from Costa Rica,[208] had just entered clinical tests with cancer patients in England.[209] Although occurring in much smaller amounts, another compound from this plant, phyllanthostatin, is also active against tumors.[210] When the National Cancer Institute combined the two in equal amounts, strong antitumor activity was found in the laboratory against a wide range of human cancers, including colon, breast, skin, lung, and ovary cancer.[211] Further work may reveal whether similar-acting compounds occur in the pitirishi.

The pitirishi (*P. niruri*) is widely recognized as a diuretic[212] used in the treatment of urinary tract infections as well as fevers.[213] In Brazil, a tea made from the whole plant is a folk treatment for painful kidneys.[214] In the Bahamas, it goes by the name hurricane weed, or gale-wind grass. The locals boil this bitter-tasting plant to make a tea to treat poor appetite, constipation, typhoid fever, and, provided the patient doesn't have an upset stomach, flu and colds.[215]

It is very often the case that folk uses cited for *P. niruri* are really for that of a close relative, *P. amarus*. Botanically, which plant is the real one used depends largely upon the area where these species occur naturally.[216] *Phyllanthus niruri* seems to prefer wet rain forests, while *P. amarus* prefers drier climes and calcium-rich soils, such as those in Miami, Florida, where *P. amarus* is an extremely common weed.[217]

Along with *P. amarus*, a common remedy in India for asthma, bronchitis, and jaundice,[218] *P. niruri* has attracted world medical attention after significantly inhibiting replication of the hepatitis B virus,[219–221] a slow-acting pathogen linked to liver cancer that is now carried by some 300 to 500 million people worldwide. As many as 40 percent of these carriers will later die of one or another consequence of the virus if they remain carriers in adulthood, when they become the persistently infected. These consequences include liver cancer, cirrhosis, and chronic hepatitis. Each year, over one million people die as a result of being long-term carriers.

The World Health Organization (WHO) expects the number of fatalities to greatly increase in the coming years because of rapid growth of populations and a lower infant mortality rate. Every year, over 50 million more are being infected. The WHO would like to see this virus eliminated in a matter of a few decades, and vaccination programs are underway to achieve their goal by the most cost-effective means.[222]

Could an herbal medicine help? That was the question posed by a group at the Fox Chase Cancer Center in Philadelphia, where a massive search of the world's herbal literature was initiated for plants used against jaundice (acute hepatitis) and other liver diseases. *Phyllanthus* turned up as one of the most promising for follow-up.[223] Clinical trials of *P. amarus* were initiated in various countries around the world, including Brazil.[224] There, as many as 3 percent now carry the virus, and in the state of Amazonas the rate is five times that.[225] With 70 percent of those twenty years old and under positive for the virus, that may be the highest rate of infection in the world. So far, the Indians in Brazil have shown the highest rates of hepatitis.[226] The hope for *Phyllanthus* is to provide an abundantly available nontoxic alternative not only to treat the disease, but ideally to render carriers sero-negative for the virus so they won't pass it on to others. Combined with vaccines, *Phyllanthus*, or perhaps other herbs combined, might make a significant contribution to the eradication of viral hepatitis. The need is urgent, especially since means of transmission are essentially the same as those for HIV.[227]

The Nobel scientist who discovered the hepatitis B vaccine, Dr. Baruch S. Blumberg, not only has given the project his full support but is one of its chief architects.[228] With carriers 200 times as likely to become liver cancer patients decades after infection, his hopes for the treatment are shared by many.[229] No side-effects have been found; however, the antihepatitis results to date have been conflicting.[230–234] This may have much to do with standardization: determining the active constituents in the herb and making sure their levels are adequate before use. In producing sero-negativity for the virus, the best results have been reported in Brazil and India, where about 60 percent of patients taking an encapsulated extract of the plant showed good results from as little as 600 mg a day.[235] In years to come, we can look forward to learning just how these herbs work.[236] Once that becomes known, the search can begin for the same action in other plants, including more promising species of *Phyllanthus*.[237, 238]

In Peru, the most common name for *P. niruri* is *chanca piedra*, meaning "shatter stone." More than one physician there has prescribed the feathery-leafed herb to cure kidney stones and gallstones, problems from which the plant takes its common name and for which the remedy is regarded infallible.[239] This herb is now available in the United States as *quebra pedra* or *chanca pedra* ("stone breaker"), the more common names in Brazil. With over 20 million people with *undiagnosed* gallstones in the United States, and about a million new cases diagnosed every year, the cost of over $5 billion to treat this digestive disease might one day inspire clinical investigations of the herb.[240] But the cost of clinical trials in the United States being what they are, I for one am not holding my breath.

LESSONS FROM A SHAMAN

The time-worn practices of Peruvian shamans are among the most enchanting while rapidly diminishing systems of healing ever uncovered in South America.[241, 242] The shamans of Peru became the subject of repeated expeditions by Colombian-born anthropologist Eduard Luis Luna. Recently, Dr. Luna learned their use of a yellow-flowered pau d'arco that Peruvians in the northeast call *tahuari* (*Tabebuia incana* A. Gentry).[243]

Dr. Luna received valuable information from Don Emilio, a shaman of Iquitos known as an *ayahuasquero* (eye-ah-whosk-arrow), whose tradition is one of the oldest and richest still available for study. As a people, ayahuasqueros are well known for remarkable abilities of memory, prophecy, telepathy, and a decidedly "holistic" approach to the treatment of disease. Don Emilio began at fourteen years old and has continued to practice for over fifty years.[244] His training was long and arduous. As with every ayahuasquero, it evolved from the use of a consciousness-altering brew made by boiling the bark of a woody vine called *ayahuasca* (*Banisteriopsis* sp.). In Quechuan, a remainder of the ancient Incan language, *ayahuasca* means "vine of the souls."[245]

The main active constituents of ayahuasca are the alkaloids harmaline and harmine, the latter originally called "telepathine."[246, 247] Ayahuasca was brought to worldwide attention in 1991 when the movie *At Play in the Fields of the Lord* featured the main character under the influence of this plant in the forests of Amazonia. Although it is seldom used outside of South America, a few psychotherapists in the United States have used the vine in therapeutic settings to facilitate insight. *Newsweek* reports that a medical doctor in New York gives ayahuasca to patients with terminal cancer to relieve their fear.[248] The vine produces strong effects and is not something to be used recreationally.

Dr. Luna learned that tahuari (*Tabebuia incana*) figures highly among the plant medicines used by ayahuasqueros as one that literally "instructs" about healing. They believe that in order for the information to be conveyed, tahuari, like other "instructors," must be ingested with ayahuasca while they abstain from sex and keep certain strict requirements of diet: mainly fish and plantains, and no salt, sugar, spices, alcohol, chicken, pork, or eggs. Tahuari is then a *doctore* or "plant teacher" and will "tell" the shaman what plants to prescribe and rituals to perform and "give" specific information on diagnoses.[249]

To the shaman Don Emilio, tahuari is "as strong as iron" and teaches "very good medicine." Dr. Luna explains: "Tahuari is supposed to be quite high in the hierarchy of *plant-teachers,* and a shaman who manipulates this plant is as strong as the tree itself."[250]

Virtually the same concept is found in the teachings of the Swiss alchemist and physician Paracelsus (1493–1541), although it is probably universal in primitive medicine. If a plant had features that in some way resembled a particular body organ, or characteristics reminiscent of a disease or other bodily condition, it became accordingly useful. This follows the ancient precept of "like curing like." For example, a plant yielding a red-colored juice might be taken to signify that it acts on the blood, while a plant that causes blisters might be applied to treat similar swellings. The concept of plant *signatures* went beyond mere physical features of a plant to include a perceived *energy* or *vital essence* that the physician would incorporate in selecting an appropriate remedy to best match the patient's symptoms.

Don Emilio regards trees as superior *doctores*, and Dr. Luna writes that shamans "who have taken very strong drugs from trees" and followed the diet are respected as being more knowledgeable. They are called *paleros*, from the Spanish *palo*: roughly, "big tree." He adds that in concept a *palero* is often associated with a kind of witch, "because the temptation to use evil powers is stronger the more is learned."[251] The idea of a witch can also be seen in the shamans of northwest Peru, who fashion magical canes ("varas") from *Tabebuia impetiginosa* and use them to cure, to gain visions, and to attack or defend against enemies. The vara is passed on as a staff of power inherited from a master shaman by a successor. The spirit of the vara may be bad or good.[252]

Following an expedition to Peru in 1984, Dr. Luna graciously responded to some of my inquiries about tahuari, which he had put to Don Emilio on my behalf. He writes:

> *Tahuari* is used in the Peruvian Amazonas first of all for diabetes. The bark is sometimes put in alcohol, and is taken as a general preventative remedy along with chuchuhuasi (*Maytenus ebenifolia*) and other trees.[253]

In her popular book *Witch Doctor's Apprentice: Hunting for Medicinal Plants in the Amazon* (New York: Citadel Press, 1990), ethnobotanist Nicole Maxwell reports that in the area of Iquitos, using the bark against cancer has not been well known; however, in controlling diabetes tahuari is "praised." Even so, other expeditionists in Peru informed her that tahuari is also used by indigenous people to treat kidney and liver ailments, and that by some tribes "startling success" was found with tahuarí against tumors. Still other reports of cancer remissions were known from the villages of Callao, San José, and Tushmo.[254]

MAYTENUS

But what was the herb called chuchuhuasi that Don Emilio combined with pau d'arco? I asked myself that question over seven years ago, and I'm still finding information about it. By that I mean that we in the North seem to have overlooked a good many studies in our pursuit of effective herbal medicines—in fact, few tropical American herbs have been the subject of so many studies.

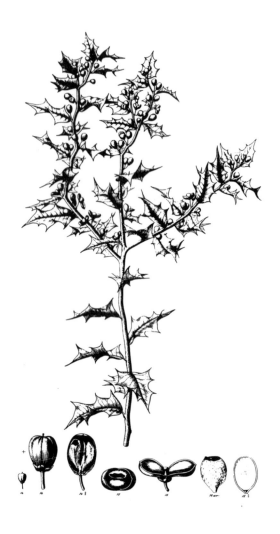

Espinheira santa (*Maytenus ilicifolia*). From Carlos F. P. De Martius and
Augustus G. Eichler, *Flora Brasiliensis, 1861–1879*, vol. 11, part 1
(Weinheim, Germany: Verlag von J. Cramer, 1967), reprint.

Maxwell had some intriguing things to say about it. In Iquitos, she found *Maytenus* taken in saloons as one of the new "jungle drinks." She reported that next to a crude alcoholic beverage made from sugar cane (aguardiente), chuchuhuasi was the most popular beverage drunk by the men who live by the rivers. This particular chuchuhuasi was identified as *Maytenus ebenifolia*. It is also likely the most widely known herbal medication in Peru, as well as Colombia. Steeped for seven days in white rum or aguardiente, the root-bark of this tree is reputedly an aphrodisiac and a cure for impotence. It is also a "general tonic" for both sexes.[255]

Maxwell witnessed restorative effects of the jungle drink firsthand in two women who were extremely weak with undiagnosed illness. She also heard reports of cancer cures from the plant and an account of someone who had been paralyzed in one arm from insecticide poisoning and had regained full motion in a few months on chuchuhuasi. She noted the lack of evidence to support such effects, including a widespread claim of the herb curing rheumatism.[256]

It was more intriguing to learn that like the shaman in Peru, who uses the bark of chuchuhuasi,[257, 258] Professor Accorsi mixed pau d'arco with a species of *Maytenus* (*M. ilicifolia* Mart.), which is commonly known in Brazil as *Espinheira santa*.[259, 260] And elsewhere in the tropics, there are reports of *Maytenus* in African folk medicine for treating excessive mucus discharge, wounds,[261] and cancer.[262]

These plants contain antibiotic compounds that in animals have shown potent antitumor and antileukemic activities at very low dosages (of micrograms per kilogram of body weight). As one of several active constituents, maytansine was first isolated from African species.[263, 264] Maytansine was tested in cancer patients in the United States during the 1970s,[265–267] but it was not considered sufficiently active to warrant further development,[268] and in the doses used it showed too much toxicity.[269] Still, a few significant regressions of cancer occurred in ovarian carcinoma and in lymphoma.[270]

In Brazil, as part of ongoing research with local herbs to find cancer treatments, earlier clinical studies found good results with the compound maytenin,[271] a quinoid triterpene derived from the roots of *Maytenus ilicifolia*.[272–274] Applied topically to treat carcinomas, it showed little irritation.[275] Other tests using the compound intravenously in patients with resistant carcinomas found best results in epidermal carcinoma (larynx, tongue base, and tonsil pillars). No toxic effects were found, but neither were there any "cures."[276] It appears that the best results are from topical uses, just as indicated by folk medicine.[277, 278]

Further clues to the activity of *Maytenus* come from studies of another species (*M. laevis* Reiss.) widely used in the Andean regions of the Amazon in Ecuador, Colombia, and Peru. Commonly known as *chuchuhuashi*, the red or golden bark of the root is used in Colombian folk medicine to treat arthritis. The trunk bark has shown anti-inflammatory activity, and the root bark contains water-soluble catechin tannins. Their presence may explain the anti-inflammatory action and protective effect against radiation shown by a water extract of the trunk bark. The triterpene maytenin (or tingenone) and a related compound (22-hydroxytingenone) also found in the bark have both shown antitumor activity.[279]

In the province of Corrientes in Argentina's northeast, the same plant occurs as a shrub called *cangorosa*, a name also referring to cancer. A leaf decoction is said to improve the skin and "to calm or avoid menstrual pains."[280] The Mexicans make a decoction of the bark of *mangle rojo* (*Maytenus phyllanthiodes* Benth.), which is used to wash wounds, to quench thirst, and to treat ulcers, stomach ache, and poor blood circulation.[281]

The bark of chuchuhuasi is famous in western Amazonia, where it is more commonly used by people in the urban centers. It seems they now regard it more highly than do the Indians in remote areas, perhaps because of the ailments they suffer and apply it to. The most common use in this region is for rheumatism. To prepare the herb for pain, the bark is soaked overnight in cane liquor, and the resulting tincture is drunk.[282]

In Colombia, the Siona Indians take a "piece of the trunk" (5 cm) and boil it in water (two liters) until the decoction reduces to half. To "cure" arthritis and rheumatism, they take "a small cupful" three times a day for a week. They also regard the decoction as a stimulant.[283]

In the lowland rain forest of eastern Ecuador, the Quijos Quichua Indians use the stem-bark of *chucchu huashu* (trembling back). A decoction of chucchu huashu (*Maytenus krukovii* A.C. Smith) is taken for rheumatism, aching muscles, menstrual aches, stomach aches, and general aching. For rheumatism, the males occasionally take the herb steeped in alcohol. For a blood-building tonic, the reddish inner bark of this species, which is described as extremely bitter, is chewed or decocted. This is given to patients recovering from tuberculosis or who display a pale complexion, and to those suffering from bronchitis, stomach ache, or fever. No limit is placed on the quantity the patient may drink, but it must be taken before breakfast for a period of one month.[284]

Records in Brazil hold that the leaves of espinheira santa (*Maytenus ilicifolia*), which appear remarkably like those of holly, are applied as an analgesic (pain reliever), an intestinal antiseptic, and a tonic.[285] Applications of the leaves include an ointment for treating skin cancer and a decoction as a wash for cancers. Other names in Brazil include *limaosinho* and *cancerosa*.[286] This is the species Professor Accorsi combined with pau d'arco.[287]

According to various herbalists in Brazil, espinheira santa is widely available and more commonly used for such problems as acne, anemia, stomach ulcers, cancer of the uterus, and constipation. Comparable activity to a well-known anti-ulcer drug (cimetidine) was shown with a water extract of two *Maytenus* species (*M. aquafolium* and *M. ilicifolia*) in animals. Gastric ulcers, chronic gastritis, and dyspepsias have long been treated with *Maytenus* in Brazilian folk medicine, but this was the first time an anti-ulcerogenic effect was demonstrated scientifically. Oral administration showed a protective effect against ulcer formation. *Maytenus* also caused an increase in gastric juices and a higher pH.[288]

Herbalists will be interested to know that even after fifteen months of storage a *Maytenus* extract remained stable,[289] and I have yet to find anyone who can recall any sign of toxicity from its use. In a commonly used laboratory test to detect mutation effects in bacteria, the leaf extract showed no mutagenicity.[290] An extensive toxicological study of the effect of *Maytenus* on rats proved that daily oral doses (3 grams of leaf powder per 150 ml of boiling water)[291]—360 times that used by people[292]—produced no toxicity.[293]

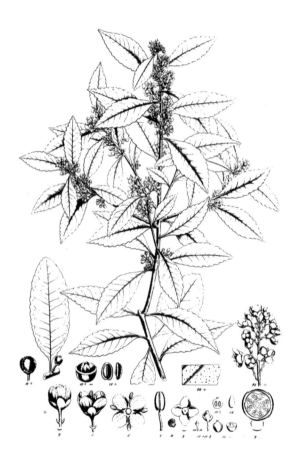

Yerba maté (*Ilex paraquayensis*). From Carlos F. P. De Martius and
Augustus G. Eichler, *Flora Brasiliensis, 1861–1879*, vol. 11, part 1.
(Weinheim, Germany: Verlag von J. Cramer, 1967), reprint.

In Paraguay, the same herb is used as a long-term contraceptive taken alone or in combination with other herbs in a contraceptive formula.[294] Because it also figures in formulas used to induce abortion,[295] this practice raises concerns of safety for pregnant women or those hoping to conceive. Testing the safety of the leaves in pregnant rats and examining their offspring, Brazilian scientists could find no signs of abnormalities. Estrus cycles were normal, and congenital defects were absent in the pups. Neither did they find adverse fertility effects in male rats.[296] I can only conclude that any claims of abortive or contraceptive effects from this herb alone appear to be without substance.

In Bolivia, Paraguay, and Uruguay, cangorosa (*Maytenus ilicifolia*) is added to the national tea, yerba maté (*Ilex paraguayensis*).[297] The leaf extract sent to me from a pharmacy in Brazil tasted sweet, something like candy licorice, but others have reported a bitter flavor. Several companies in the United States now carry *Maytenus* extract which is expected to become more widely available in the years ahead.

Generally, herbs from the tropics are more flavorful than those in our temperate climate, and I expect this appeal will hasten their arrival. Pau d'arco tea reminds me of cinnamon.

FOUR

Inside Pau d'Arco

Pau d'arco is today one of the most widely used immunostimulating plants known. But it was a long time in becoming so regarded. Until all the commotion caused by the media in Brazil, there were few studies on the activity of the bark. Then suddenly, that situation changed.

COMMISSION OF INQUIRY

Immediately after prescription of the bark in Brazilian hospitals was banned, the Secretary of Health for the state of São Paulo appointed a commission to investigate pau d'arco, *and all related information*.[1] A seminar was organized by Brazil's Academy of Pharmacy in the spring of 1967, just weeks after the news appeared in *O'Cruzeiro*. Experts in botany, chemistry, and pharmacology gathered to share their views, that others might find them helpful in the colossal task of a pau d'arco investigation. A search of the literature found that information on the medicinal uses of the tree remained scarce, scattered, and lacking objective results: Pau d'arco of practically every flower color were mentioned as useful, "especially in syphilis and its manifestations." Dr. Osvaldo A. Costa proposed that since ulcers of the skin were once thought to be syphilis, "among these there must have existed the [abnormal growths] we now identify [as tumors]."[2] But apart from this one reasonable assumption, in the end the commission found only inconclusive results.

A respected Brazilian botanist, Dr. Theodore Peckholt, was of the firm opinion that pau d'arco deserved serious study. He thought it odd for the director of the National Cancer Society to declare no interest in pau d'arco, to say that the society had better things to do than to "waste its time with tomfoolery."[3] However, aside from all this neglect, what followed was a number of attempts to isolate pau d'arco's active components and to determine the threat of toxicity. The safety of pau d'arco is discussed in "Looking for Toxicity," page 97.

COMPOUND CURIOSITY

Searching for pau d'arco's therapeutic activities, the São Paulo Institute of Biology turned up no significant pain-relieving or sedative actions, either from the "alkaloidal" portion of the bark or the whole-bark extract.[4] The term *alkaloid* is applied to a wide assortment of usually bitter-tasting compounds from the plant kingdom. Often, they show powerful actions in animals and in humans. There are numerous examples. The antimalarial "quinine" from Peruvian bark (*Cinchona* sp.), still found in tonic water, is being applauded as the starter compound for a drug alternative to cortico-steroids for the treatment of rheumatoid arthritis.[5] Caffeine is an alkaloid we all know from *Coffea* species, and morphine is one we know from poppy plants (*Papaver* sp.), so you can see why the interest in pau d'arco's alkaloids.

In one study, rats were injected with saponins from the bark (*T. impetiginosa*).[6] Saponins take their name from the Latin *sapo*, meaning "soap." You can get some indication of the saponin content in an herbal tea by shaking it up and down and watching for the amount or lack of foam produced. In certain plants, in which the content of saponin is high, the term *soap* becomes more literal. For example, the barks of *Quillaja* species hold so much saponin that many of the natives in South America store these barks dried and later use them with water to clean laundry. Because the saponins in soapbark inhibit fungi,[7] this plant is especially useful in tropical South America, for there fungi are constantly attacking fabric and causing difficult-to-treat infections in people. In Peru, the soapbark tree (*Q. saponaria*) also finds use in cleaning hair, head, and mouth, but internal use must be avoided, for it is also a cardiac depressant.[8]

Taken internally, many saponins are generally known to produce stomach upset and diarrhea, depending, of course, upon the amount consumed and the interaction of other naturally occurring constituents of the saponin-containing plant consumed.[9] University of São Paulo pharmacologists Seizi Oga and Tomhiko Sekino concluded from saponins in the bark of pau d'arco (*T. impetiginosa*) that the level of "tolerance shown by the rats to doses considered sufficiently high, demonstrated the low toxicity of the extract."[10] Saponins can also increase the availability of active constituents in herbs by increasing their solubility in water, and by enhancing their digestive tract absorption.[11]

Some scientists in Brazil wondered whether the "unusual increase" in pau d'arco's use in popular medicine, especially against cancer, might be

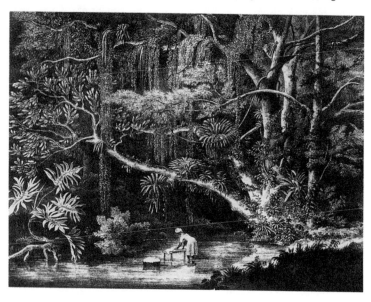

A laundromat in the jungles of Ubatuba, province of Rio de Janeiro, 1840–1906. From Carlos F. P. De Martius and Augustus G. Eichler, *Flora Brasiliensis, 1840–1906,* vol. 1, part 1 (Weinheim, Germany: Verlag von J. Cramer, 1965), reprint.

due to radioactivity. That question was pursued in 1967 by researchers at the Institute of Geography and Geology, who found that in spite of "innumerable therapeutic virtues attributed to it," the bark (*T. heptaphylla*) had no radioactive elements whatsoever. What they did find was a high average content (1.9 percent) of nonradioactive strontium, an element closely related to calcium and used in toothpastes for people with sensitive teeth.[12]

By 1969, studies on the bark ceased to appear in Brazil. For many it seemed that the phenomenon of pau d'arco had finally reached some rational end. Brazilian scientists had conducted tests with rodents for signs of antitumor activity, but any activity they found was at best weak.[13, 14] An outstanding authority on the chemistry of Brazilian plants, Dr. Walter B. Mors, recalls the dominating opinion at the time was that oft-claimed therapeutic effects could not be rationally explained.[15] Much the same message was reflected by the Brazilian Cancer Society as recently as 1983. They admitted that *some* physicians still used the tea, but as far as the society was concerned, claims of the 1960s were "strongly" disputed.[16] Nevertheless, in more recent years Brazilian interest in the bark has been cropping up again, in both the marketplace and university laboratories.

SIGNS OF IMMUNOSTIMULATION

Despite the lack of test results showing a reason for pau d'arco's activity against disease, the normalization of blood cell counts was repeatedly witnessed by South American physicians who examined cancer patients on pau d'arco. At the Municipal Hospital of Santo André, a case was recorded in which the white blood cell count in a patient with advanced leukemia normalized after only four weeks' treatment with the bark.[17] And in Cordoba, Argentina, a woman diagnosed with acute lymphocytic leukemia had shown dramatic improvement in her blood in a matter of days.[18]

Teodoro Meyer referred to "curable" illnesses becoming established in the body through poor food, malnutrition, "and the lack of organic defenses." Liver ailments, anemia, asthma, diabetes, cystitis, rheumatism, and prostatitis, he wrote, are among the curable illnesses that are "fully treatable and curable, allowing a combined treatment" with his elixir (see chapter 1) added to the medication prescribed. When it came to "incurable" diseases, and he included leukemia and cancer, Meyer reasoned that the majority of patients would have to continue the treatment for a very long time—for most, the duration of their lives. He advised the treatment "be lengthy, uninterrupted and maintained at a minimum useful dosage."[19] With those words he inadvertently referred to the character of most immunostimulants. Drs. Hildebert Wagner and A. Proksch of the Institute of Pharmaceutical Biology at the University of Munich explain that these are largely compounds that act in a "*nonspecific*" way, and although stimulating "defenses" of the immune system, they're not like vaccines: "their pharmacological efficacy fades comparatively quickly," thus requiring administration on a continuous basis or in intervals.[20]

Meyer further claimed that the bark preparation served as an aid in reducing "counter-reactions to medicines and specifically to antibiotics." But in what could be interpreted his most obvious reference to immunostimulation, Meyer wrote, "In its broad action, it puts the body in a defensive posture, giving it the energy it needs to defend itself and to resist disease."[21] The same actions describe the typical *fu-zheng* herbs used in traditional Chinese medicine, many of which are now known to have significant effects on the immune system. Fu-zheng herbs are applied in treatments of cancer to decrease the untoward effects of medicines, strengthen the resistance of patients, protect bodily functions, and "increase the curative effect of the drug used."[22]

PAU D'ARCO COMES TO NEW JERSEY

Odd as it may seem today, the first published report of pau d'arco stimulating immune cell activity was the work of F. J. DiCarlo and team at the Warner-Lambert Research Institute in Morris Plains, New Jersey, in 1963. This is the same company that brought us Rolaids and Listerine. Coincidentally, *Maytenus* showed up in their study, too.[23]

Samples of pau d'arco and *Maytenus*, as well as other plants, were tested in mice to see if they would accelerate *phagocytosis*, which is the cell-engulfing or "eating" ability of phagocytic immune cells, such as the macrophage. Collectively, their results indicated that plant sources of immunostimulants are more common than might be supposed. No mention was made of taking their selections from folk medicine, yet half of some twenty-four plants stimulated phagocytic activity to various degrees.[24]

The pau d'arco tested in this study (*Tabebuia barbata* [E. Mey.] Sandw.) occurs in the lowland regions of the Venezuelan and Brazilian Amazon with beautiful yellow-throated magenta flowers.[25] Common names in Brazil include *pau d'arco roxo*, *tauary do gapo*, *ipé roxo*, *pau d'arco*, and *capitari*. This pau d'arco is mostly found in the heart of Amazonia, along the Río Orinoco upper regions bordering Colombia.[26] In Colombian folk medicine, the bark of this tree is said to have some sort of toxic action, but it is still employed. A decoction is used for bathing the skin to treat epidermal diseases, such as pimples and ulcers.[27] The Kuripakos Indians of eastern Colombia make a decoction of the leaves for a tea to relieve flatulence after a meal of tapir meat,[28] and in the State of Pará in northern Brazil, the bark of this tree (*pau d'arco-da-beira* meaning "pau d'arco of the shore") is boiled to make a tea taken for "vaginal excretions."[29]

The leaves were also tested and appear to be five times more potent than the bark; however, the immunostimulating activity of this pau d'arco, whether of the bark or of the leaves, was not statistically significant. In all of twenty-four different plants, greatest activity was found with *Maytenus laevis*, an evergreen from Venezuela. An injection (intravenous) of the leaf-suspension showed eight times the potency of the pau d'arco bark.[30]

Although the leaves of *Maytenus* became the main subject of the investigation, with oral administration the results showed activity the researchers could only describe as "erratic" and "inconsistent." Nevertheless, DiCarlo and team regarded the erratic activity of the leaves as "unique" and worthy of further investigation.[31]

DISCOVERIES IN HAWAII

The bark became the subject of a deeper immunologic investigation in the United States in 1984 and again in 1985, partly as the result of its local popularity. This work was conducted by Dr. Y. Hokama, head of the Department of Pathology at the John A. Burns School of Medicine of the University of Hawaii at Manoa.[32] My interview with him in 1985 revealed that he was typical of scientists of Asian descent, who regard plants as worthy leads in the discovery of new agents to combat disease.

Hokama related that he had been looking for a subject his students could work on as part of their graduate program. Pau d'arco became an enticing candidate when he learned that there were a number of calls to the university from people hoping to learn something definite about a bark tea from Brazil that was reputedly useful in the treatment of cancer and a long list of other diseases. Just as on the mainland, accounts of "cures" circulated in the Islands, one of them concerning a man who had been diagnosed with advanced cancer of the prostate and told that his condition was beyond treatment. With Hokama's own curiosity and no lack of interest from his students, a supply of pau d'arco was obtained for initial antitumor studies as a fascinating if not challenging project for a few seniors working toward graduation.[33]

Initially, they tested a commercial pau d'arco "extract" obtained at a local health food store. But finding it devoid of antitumor activity, they ended up using water extracts prepared like the tea. They made their tea much according to the instructions on the box: about four tablespoons of bark boiled in four to five cups of water. For dosage they used an amount about equivalent to the four or five cups a day suggested. The tea proved remarkably nontoxic in mice, with doses of up to 2,000 mg/kg very well tolerated. The pau d'arco they used was identified as *Tabebuia heptaphylla*, a purple pau d'arco with a reddish brown inner bark.[34–37]

Their results were most promising—especially to anyone in search of cancer inhibitors for the diet. Hokama and students concluded that the bark may protect against the migration (metastases) of some tumors, since they observed less incidence of tumors (Lewis lung carcinoma) in mice treated with the bark; however, growth of the primary tumor was not suppressed.[38] In other words, there were no cures. But the fact that the bark protected mice insofar as it kept the lung cancer from migrating is not without significance, for once tumor cells stop spreading throughout the system, the patient stands a better chance of survival and success from what other treatments may be used to finally eradicate the cancer.

Was the tumor inhibition somehow the result of immunostimulation? That was the question posed by David H. Moikeha, Jr., and Dr. Hokama in a follow-up study. In order to obtain an indication of this activity, they used the same bark in cell cultures of macrophages from mice. This time the tea was made using ten grams of bark (about six tablespoons) boiled in seventy-five ml of water for forty-five minutes. Their results showed that the bark had significantly stimulated macrophages and that that activity was increased with each increased dose until the maximum stimulation at the highest dose tested (5 mg pau d'arco/ml of the macrophage suspension).[39]

The work didn't stop there. They decided a new antitumor study was needed and were able to test a different species of pau d'arco with a donation of bark (*T. impetiginosa*) collected from the estate of the botanist Teodoro Meyer in northwest Argentina.[40] For dosage, they followed the same close adherence to "suggested" amounts of pau d'arco from the box of Brazilian bark. But this time they examined the post-surgical effect of pau d'arco in mice with lung cancer. They wanted to see what effect the bark would have on the survival of mice, knowing that even though they had eliminated the main tumor with surgery, some cancer cells would remain and by their very nature would "metastasize" or migrate to the lungs.[41]

A day after surgery the mice began treatment. Every second day for a month they received stomach injections of pau d'arco (166.65 mg per kilo of body weight, or mg/kg). When fifty days from the time of surgery they examined the mice for tumors, the results were most impressive. Moikeha and Hokama found a "highly significant inhibition of metastases to the lung," with no growth of the cancer visible in the lungs of any survivors. Eighty percent of the mice without the bark had died, but for those that received the bark 71 percent had survived and looked fine.[42]

The Hawaiian researchers left inspiring remarks for others who might follow in the study of pau d'arco:

New approaches to eradicate the few tumor cells that resist conventional therapies involve those which explore the possibility of general antineoplastic activity in organic extracts. This study, as well as others, suggests that appropriately activated macrophages provide a biological approach to the destruction of the few, but fatal, tumor cells that resist or escape conventional therapies. The exhibition of such activity in the aqueous extracts of the *Tabebuia* has potential significance, since people can drink this agent as tea.[43]

ANSWERS FROM MUNICH: QUINONES

After several years investigating the bark, Dr. Hildebert Wagner, head of the Institute for Pharmaceutical Biology at the University of Munich in Germany, found reason to suspect that some if not much of pau d'arco's reputation in folk medicine had its basis in immunostimulation.[44] After testing various pau d'arco barks, Dr. Wagner established that they hold a "good" level of immunomodulating activity.[45] The bark of *T. impetiginosa* enhanced the *cell-eating* or phagocytic action of isolated immune cells by 40 percent.[46] Larger doses were *less* immunostimulating than smaller ones, which is typical of immunostimulants.[47]

Lower versus higher doses and concentrations of pau d'arco were also more effective in antitumor studies reported by the U.S. National Cancer Institute as early as 1962. And in contrast to what Brazilian tests were showing around the same time,[48] some of the NCI tests showed significant levels of antitumor activity.[49–54]

When a water extract of the bark (*T. heptaphylla*) was injected (250 mg/kg) into the lining surrounding the abdominal area (peritoneum) of tumor-bearing mice, there was a 65 percent reduction in Sarcoma 180 tumor size compared to controls not treated with the bark, and five out of six mice survived. With another of the main species of pau d'arco used in Brazil, a water extract of *Tabebuia roseo-alba* (incorrectly *Tecoma odontodiscus* in the NCI study),[55] there was a 66 percent tumor inhibition rate (from 125 mg/kg) and six out of six mice survived.[56] Doubling and quadrupling those doses and using inherently more concentrated alcoholic extracts, inhibition rates dropped to 39 percent and less.[57] Of course, at that time effects on the immune system were not something the NCI had much interest in, especially from plants, and the results were readily discounted as inconsistent. As for why the Brazilian tests had turned up negligible antitumor activity with the same test procedures, variations in the levels of active constituents due to seasonal changes, storage, or harvesting factors is the most likely explanation.

Drs. Hokama and Wagner both considered what kind of substance might be responsible for the immunostimulation displayed by the bark. Both suspected biological pigments known as quinones.[58] Although quinones are found throughout nature, biochemists regard them as being of extreme importance. This is because the quinones are primarily involved in the biological transfer of hydrogen and of electrons. Because of their ability to shuttle electrons in cellular respiration, they have the distinction of functioning as "electron transformers." Their "catalytic" character in the transport of electrons is found in their structure, which allows them to easily oxidize and reduce. Quinones serve catalytically in processes of oxidative metabolism in plants, animals, and microorganisms. There is much attention to quinones these days, as biochemists are now recognizing their presence as important determining factors in the antioxidant and pro-oxidant status of normal and diseased cells.[59,60]

Some quinones, such as adriamycin, are applied in high doses in chemotherapy. Unfortunately, these are often toxic to healthy cells, and cells of the immune system are no exception. Still other types of quinones are causing excitement in the anti-aging arena. That is because quinones that naturally occur in our bodies operate in some very strategic places, such as the brain and connective tissue. One, called ortho-dopamine quinone, is formed in our nervous system from dopamine,[61] a neurotransmitter, and ubiquinone is an antioxidant that increases in content in skeletal muscles during intensive exercise.[62]

The possibility that quinones may play a protective role is being hotly pursued in Japan, where scientists are hoping to tap their potential in keeping the brain young and alert. A semisynthetic quinone called idebenone showed a stabilizing effect on liver cell membranes.[63] It also protected animals against liver damage due to poisons, and in elderly patients with mental impairment, it decreased dementia. Some of the latter showed fewer emotional problems. Under the trade name Avan, this quinone is now used to enhance the energy metabolism of the brain in dementia and Alzheimer's.[64] Clinical trials with this quinoidal drug are going on all over the world, and good results are being found in elderly patients with dementia, cognitive decline, and degenerative brain disorders.[65-68] Idebenone traps electrons and functions as a free radical scavenger to protect cell membranes from oxidation.[69] For that reason, it might be called a kind of "rust inhibitor" for the brain.

Some quinones appear so essential to normal functioning that researchers are wondering whether a number of these biological pigments might even be vitamins.[70] Phylloquinone is already a vitamin. Also known as vitamin K, it keeps our blood from becoming too thin by maintaining a normal blood-clotting time. Vitamin K regulates the body's synthesis of clotting factors such as prothrombin. It is interesting to note that vitamin K also plays an essential role in processes of photosynthesis.[71] Vitamin K_2 (menaquinone-1) occurs in the heartwood of pau d'arco (*T. impetiginosa*)[72] while vitamin K_3 (menadione, a synthetic derivative of vitamin K) is a potent antioxidant even in minute concentrations.[73] This is in contrast to the various oxidative quinones used in chemotherapy to literally oxidize tumor cells.

At your local health food store, you may have seen ubiquinone or coenzyme Q_{10} (CoQ), a nontoxic quinone that idebenone was originally derived from.[74] Ubiquinone boosts the activity of macrophages,[75-77] strengthens and protects the cardiovascular system and heart,[78, 79] normalizes excessive blood pressure, and reverses periodontal disease.[80] In Japan and Italy, this substance is a prescription drug for preventing muscle tissue damage from oxygen deficiency, and it is also prescribed to prevent toxic effects on the heart that result from certain anticancer and cardiac drugs.[81]

Ubiquinone, as its name implies, is ubiquitous, occurring in our bodies and throughout nature, although in minute amounts. Unlike the inherently toxic quinones, ubiquinone and related quinones are immunologically active when taken in large amounts.[82, 83] Ubiquinone is now derived from microorganisms but was at one time very expensive; it had to be taken from beef hearts or semisynthesized from an incomplete form found in tobacco plants.[84] Many informative books are available on this important substance for every level of reader.

In the world of plant-derived quinones, lawsone imparts the hair-dyeing substance in henna (*Lawsonia inermis*), and the weakly antifungal juglone in green walnut shells and leaves (*Juglans* sp.) stains skin and dyes wool a dark yellowish brown. Because juglone and lawsone inhibit skin damage caused by UV rays and serve as self-tanning agents, extracts of green walnut shells and henna leaves are widely used in European tanning creams.[85, 86] The laxative quinone emodin found in the leaves of *Aloe* plants[87] and the cardioactive tanshinones I and II from the root of red sage, or tan-shen (*Salvia miltorrhiza* Bunge), are among the better-known herbal sources of quinones. Tanshinones inhibit the aggregation of blood platelets, which can lead to clots, increase the flow of blood in the heart, and reduce the oxygen demand of the heart.[88] A semisynthetic form of tanshinone II is used in China to treat cerebral thromboembolism (blood vessels clogged with aggregated blood) and cardiovascular diseases.[89]

Before Dr. Wagner's discoveries, similar quinones to those in the heart-wood of yellow[90]and purple pau d'arco[91]were already found immuno-stimulating by researchers at the Institute of Microbiology of the Czecho-slovak Academy of Sciences in 1981. What they found was that many simple naturally occurring quinones and their derivatives are *immuno-suppressive*, while still others are *immunostimulating*. Typically, larger doses are *suppressive* or even toxic, and small doses are either *inactive* or *immunostimulating* (macrophages, B-cells, and T-cells).[92]

In Germany, Dr. Wagner and colleagues investigated the effects of high and low concentrations of quinones from several plants, as well as extracts of the plants themselves. In test tube experiments, human immune cells responded to higher concentrations (1 mg to 100th of a mg/ml of cells) with immunosuppressive or cytotoxic results, whereas low concentrations "showed in nearly all cases immunostimulating proper-ties."[93] By "low" Dr. Wagner means incredibly small concentrations of quinones: as much as *100 millionths of a millionth of a gram* and as little as *ten 1,000ths of a millionth of a millionth of a gram*![94] A methanolic extract of the inner bark (*T. impetiginosa*) caused a 25 percent enhancement of macrophage activity (phagocytosis) from only *one millionth of a millionth of a gram* of the extract (per ml of cells), or one picogram.[95] And yet, using a water extract, the same concentration of bark produced a 48.3 percent rate of stimulation.[96] Activity from minute doses occurred not only with pau d'arco (*T. heptaphylla* and *T. impetiginosa*), but also with other plants used in complementary medicine to treat cancer, such as the carnivorous Venus's-flytrap (*Dionaea muscipula*) and another carnivore, a kind of sundew (*Drosera ramentacea*) native to Madagascar.[97]

In the quest to uncover medicinally active plants and plant derivatives, Dr. Wagner concludes that an immunostimulating effect with such very small amounts of otherwise cytotoxic substances "can explain a variety of observed antiviral and antitumoral effects of plant extracts . . . for which a direct cytotoxicity could be ruled out."[98] These findings with pau d'arco[99] are likely to be pertinent to other quinone-containing plants used to treat cancer, such as Venus's-flytrap,[100] and this possibility has been the subject of much ongoing research.[101–103]

CRYSTALS IN THE WOOD

So far in work with pau d'arco bark, scientists know the identity of more than one immuno-active quinone.[104, 105] One of these, called lapachol,[106] was much earlier named after the lapacho or pau d'arco tree.

Early in this century in Brazil, Yale University foresters Samuel J. Record and Clayton D. Mell reported that they had found numerous species of *Tabebuia* in the tropical American rain forests. The tree was accredited with "astringent" bark, valued as a treatment for syphilis. Record and Mell used local names to classify the different woods, giving pau d'arco to a group having wood of an "oily olive-brown color" and vessels containing a "yellow crystaline" matter visible on the wood surface and appearing like sulfur.[107] This crystalline matter—in its pure form a bright, almost iridescent, yellow—is the biologically active plant pigment lapachol. It can be scraped from the planed wood, where in its raw state it appears duller and darker, much like curry powder.

At the Recife Institute of Antibiotics in Pernambuco, Brazil, Dr. Oswaldo Goncalves De Lima began over thirty years of research with this quinone after discovering that it held some interesting and potentially valuable medicinal properties.[108] Studies at the institute (now a World Health Organization center for medicinal plant research) have more recently found that lapachol has antiviral activity against herpes simplex types I and II,[109] poliovirus type I, a number of influenza viruses, and several others.[110] Naturally, more work would be necessary in order to learn whether lapachol could be used to treat the diseases these viruses cause.

Nature didn't restrict lapachol to pau d'arco. At Banaras University in Varanasi, India, R. K. Goel and colleagues found the quinone in experiments with an extract of teak bark and wood (*Tectona grandis* L., family Verbenaceae). The extract proved active against peptic ulcers, one of the uses herbalists make of teak in India. The therapeutic effect on ulcers in guinea pigs and rats was significant. Goel subsequently worked with the powdered roots and found lapachol. When ingested by animals (5 mg/ kg) it was effective in reversing aspirin-induced ulcers. As a preventive agent, lapachol provided significant protection against duodenal ulcers and against stress-induced gastric ulcers. The quinone provided five times the potency of the wood chip and bark extract.[111]

An anti-inflammatory action from lapachol has also been observed in humans,[112] an effect that may be due to an inhibitory action on overactive immune cells,[113] or other mediators of inflammation in the body, such as prostaglandins—fatty acids that regulate acid secretion in the stomach, control inflammatory processes, and perform a host of other primary functions. In experiments with rats, the Federal University of Pernambuco in Recife, Brazil, found that taken orally, lapachol was a more potent anti-inflammatory than phenylbutazone—at inhibiting both the swelling due to inflammation (edema) and the formation of abcesses.[114] The Department of Antibiotics at the university is currently formulating a topical anti-inflammatory preparation of lapachol.[115]

Currently in Brazil, lapachol is made (synthesized) for oral ingestion[116]— its most effective route[117]—as a cancer therapeutic used in combination with other medicines or by itself.[118] Dosages at the Cancer Hospital in

Recife typically reach two grams a day. So far, the only cancer patients to receive the drug have been the terminally ill with conditions so advanced they were resistant to all other therapies.[119] In terminal conditions it isn't unusual for experimental drugs to be used as a last resort.

The results in Brazil, however early,[120] are in contrast to the complete abandonment of lapachol by the U.S. National Cancer Institute (NCI). Lapachol was once a very promising compound. Although chemically related to some quinone anticancer drugs already in use, such as adriamycin, lapachol showed considerably less toxicity. But when the NCI tested lapachol in 1967, "for 5 days," researchers found it unsuccessful against leukemia (chronic myelocytic): patients' conditions either remained the same or grew worse.[121, 122] The outcome was by most accounts regrettable. It came after years of testing in animals in which lapachol proved only mildly toxic and had shown "highly significant" activity against an implanted tumor cell line (Walker 256)[123] used to test potential new drugs, but that has since been abandoned by the NCI for being a poor predictor of activity.[124]

Brazilian scientists have found that when terminal cancer patients are given lapachol, pain is often reduced or eliminated altogether; however, in five of eight patients, tumors regressed either temporarily or not at all. But even with those terminal cases, three patients remained alive and later found their cancer in remission. One had kidney cancer (adenocarcinoma); another, cancer of the mouth (carcinoma); and a third patient had stomach cancer (adenocarcinoma of the abdomen and large intestine). Length of treatment ranged from a matter of months to as long as two years in the case of the stomach cancer.[125] In the hope of developing an intravenous formula and of achieving thereby, higher levels in the blood, more recent work has focused on improving the solubility of lapachol, which would allow it to be injected.[126] Yet, however mildly toxic for an anticancer quinone, lapachol still can't be used during pregnancy.[127]

The herbalist will be more interested to learn that the NCI came to test lapachol not through pau d'arco, but through a distant cousin of the same plant family (Bignoniaceae). At a meeting of the American Association for Cancer Research in April 1967, it was announced that root extracts of an East Indian plant called the patala (*Stereospermum suaveolens* D.C.) had shown "reproducible activity" against cancer in rats. Lapachol was found to be the compound responsible.[128]

Folklore records tell us that the root of the patala has been used in the treatment of abdominal tumors and nasal polyps (a growth protruding from the mucous membrane of the nose). Preparations include clarified butter (ghee), enemas, and powder.[129] The patala is widely distributed in India, and its various parts are used in a variety of diseases. The bark of the root is an ingredient of the Indian tonic *dasmula*, while the flowers are made into a confection taken as an aphrodisiac.[130] As a post-abortion treatment, a decoction of the patala is used to prepare rice, which is eaten to relieve pain and stiffness and to cleanse the uterus.[131] A close relative, the pink-flowered *S. chelonoides* is used in Ayurvedic medicine to treat "nerve disorders."[132]

WHAT ABOUT THE WOOD?

Less well known outside of South America is that in addition to the bark, some doctors employing complementary medicines use an extract of the heartwood.[133–135] In Argentina, the bark and wood of the *lapacho rosado* (*T. impetiginosa*), whether boiled or steeped, has been applied in popular medicine to treat diseases of the bladder and kidney.[136] Experiments in Brazil found an alcoholic extract of the heartwood produced more than twice the antitumor effect (80 percent inhibition) that a water extract of the bark produced, and from less than half the dose (150 mg/kg).[137] Professor Accorsi informs me that doctors using natural treatments believe that the heartwood extract works best of all.[138] Dr. Fadlo Fraige Filho, former clinical director of the Municipal Hospital of Santo André, expressed the same view. He cautioned, however, that doctors do not regard the heartwood as a panacea; the results, although reportedly "good," are not from carefully controlled clinical trials. His feeling is that when pau d'arco is used in combination with conventional treatments, perhaps including other medicinal plants, we may one day discover an effective therapy for cancer.[139]

In the timber trade, allergic reactions from pau d'arco sawdust are common. Exposure to the dust of pau d'arco woods produces irritations varying from an itchy reddening to acute dermatitis, systemic toxicity, and irritation to the respiratory tract,[140–142] reasons enough, one would think, to wonder how the wood could be used medicinally at all, at least not without *some* side-effects. When I inquired of Professor Accorsi about toxicity from the wood, he wrote that "excessive use" of the heartwood extract causes a "slight itchiness of the skin,"[143] which is the same effect too much of the bark produces.[144] When asked about side-effects from the heartwood extract, Dr. Fraige could tell me only that he knew doctors and patients who used it against cancer, and he was not aware of any undesirable effects.[145]

In a clinical study, allergic reactions of the kind the sawdust produces were not found from the extract. The Recife Institute of Antibiotics reported *no side-effects* from the "wood" (*T. impetiginosa*) in the form of a bicarbonated extract (alcoholic with a pH of 6.0), despite its application intravaginally against chronic cervicitis and cervicovaginitis (inflammation of the cervix and the cervix and vagina, respectively). That study was conceived as part of a program to investigate affordable treatments for common problems affecting the underprivileged in Brazil, accustomed to using folk medicines. Out of the multitude of herbs available, the institute chose to begin their program with pau d'arco. They noted that the bark was mentioned in Brazilian records from the late 1800s as useful in treating rheumatic, venereal, and "especially skin problems" (eczema, mange caused by mites, and herpes), as well as in the treatment of ulcers and fevers.[146]

Twenty patients used tampons that had been soaked in the wood extract, replacing them with freshly treated tampons every twenty-four hours. Treatment periods usually ranged from eight to twenty-eight days. Others douched with the extract for over a month. Yet, in all of twenty patients not a single side-effect was noticed, and all who completed the treatment had successful results. The doctors found that in some patients *Candida albicans* and *Trichomonas vaginallis* were associated with the problems treated.[147]

Even though lapachol has no effect on the vaginal cell cycle and is not absorbed systemically by this route of administration,[148] the high content of lapachol in the wood (3–4 percent)[149] alone could account for the anti-inflammatory,[150] antifungal,[151] and antibacterial[152] effects of the extract. But there are other constituents in the wood, even aside from antifungal quinones related to lapachol, that have to be considered; para-hydroxybenzoic acid, salicylic acid, quercetin,[153] and tannic acid (12.2–17.8 percent) in the wood of this pau d'arco (*T. impetiginosa*)[154] must all be playing a role.

In 1993, the December 17 issue of *Science* carried an article by researchers at the State University of New Jersey in which they showed how salicylic acid is produced in plants as part of an immune response to fight infections and also acts as a signal to activate the plants' defenses against plant pathogens such as bacteria and viruses.

Until being made into aspirin, salicylic acid (2-hydroxybenzoic acid) was once widely used for its antiseptic and food-preserving actions.[155] *Para*-hydroxybenzoic acid, an intestinal antiseptic, is antifungal, as is benzoic acid itself. Combined with salicylic acid, it was once found in drugstores as a topical antifungal preparation.[156] *Para*-hydroxybenzoic acid strongly inhibits the activity of tyrosinase,[157] an enzyme that causes pigmentation of the skin through the oxidation of tyrosine, in turn producing melanins.[158] The black of black melanoma—a deadly kind of cancer—is due to the same enzyme. Although they provide protection from ultra-violet rays,[159] melanin-containing tissues have a higher binding affinity for toxic compounds[160] and can cause cell damage from being "overloaded" with too many free radicals, industrial chemicals, some kinds of prescription drugs, herbicides, pesticides, heavy metals, or ultraviolet light.[161]

Grapes (*Vitis fructus*) are listed among the plants in ancient Chinese texts for the treatment of facial diseases. They have a very high level of activity against tyrosinase, and this is largely (71 percent) due to *para*-hydroxybenzoic acid.[162] Along with tissue-contracting catechins, this factor may partly explain the practice among tropical Asian herbalists of applying the juice of a grape plant (*Vitis compressa*) to wounds to speed healing.[163]

Long known to Arabian alchemists, benzoic acid was derived from the fragrant gum of a tree (*Styrax benzoin* Dryander) found in Sumatra. The antiseptic, diuretic, and expectorant gum was once widely used in perfumes and for centuries was regarded as a kind of frankincense.[164] There was extensive use of benzoic acid during the nineteenth century. Among diverse applications, the acid was used in bronchitis (as an expectorant), cystitis, and arthritis.[165] The main therapeutic use is in topical antiseptics for desloughing and cleansing ulcerations and wounds. Benzoic acid is also used to treat skin diseases and ringworm affecting the scalp.[166] In these applications and in its use as a nontoxic bactericidal in many kinds of packaged foods, the action is similar to that of salicylic acid.[167] In Europe, benzoic and salicylic acids are approved as additives to cosmetics to inhibit the growth of microorganisms,[168] and salicylic acid is one of the main components of a skin-cleansing formula for the face that removes dead skin cells without irritating the skin.[169]

A number of benzoic acids are also found in the bark[170] and leaves of pau d'arco and undoubtedly play a significant role in the many topical applications found in folk medicine. In the leaves, these include *para*-hydroxybenzoic, vanillic, genistic, and caffeic acids.[171]

Quercetin, also found in the wood, is available in most health food stores as a bioflavonoid (a biologically active flavonoid). Quercetin is a potent anti-inflammatory substance and local pain reliever related chemically to the histamine release-inhibitor cromolyn, an antiasthmatic drug.[172] Quercetin has shown strong antihistamine release activity in cells exposed to allergens, but not to inactivated cells.[173] By inhibiting prostaglandin synthesis and by exerting a morphinelike action at inhibiting the release of acetylcholine, it has been proposed that quercetin and quercetin-rich herbs may be useful in the treatment of acute diarrheal disease. Worldwide, this illness killed about 4.6 million children in 1980 alone, most of them less than two years old. In Asia, Africa, and Latin American countries in the same year, about 744 million children suffered acute episodes of the disease.[174]

Quercetin doubled the antileukemic activity of a drug (busulphan) used to treat chronic myeloid leukemia and may one day prove useful combined with chemotherapy.[175] Indeed, antitumor and antiviral mechanisms for this bioflavonoid have been the subject of studies worldwide for many years.[176–181] Because of potential anticarcinogenic activity, levels of quercetin in the diet from fruits, vegetables, and teas are of great interest.[182] In the Netherlands, quercetin accounted for 70 percent of the total flavonoid intake from foods, which was largely (48 percent) from tea.[183] Quercetin also occurs in the leaves of pau d'arco.[184]

Then there's tannic acid. In Britain, fungal infections of the toes and fingernails were once treated with a tannin-rich proprietary formula called Phytex. It was a paint consisting mainly of tannic acid and boric acids, salicylic acid (9 percent), hydroxybenzoate (0.35 percent), and other natural products.[185] The combination of these substances alone might explain the use of the wood extract in folk treatments of cancer, but the most active parts are still quinones, especially lapachol.

BETA-LAPACHONE

Beta-lapachone is a quinone found in the woods of various pau d'arco in smaller quantities than lapachol.[186, 187] In early tests with tumor-bearing rodents, *beta*-lapachone proved weakly active.[188] Now synthesized, *beta*-lapachone was first derived from the wood of pau d'arco in northeast Brazil, where it was initially studied for antitumor activity during the late 1960s. It has since gone on to be the subject of studies in Europe and the United States, where the interest in antiviral[189] and antitumor[190] mechanisms has focused on interrupting the DNA of pathogenic cells. For example, *beta*-lapachone blocks the replication ability of HIV, whether cells have been acutely or chronically infected by the virus. Unlike azidothymidine (AZT), which is commonly prescribed for AIDS and inhibits reproduction of HIV, the quinone appears to block the viral "long terminal repeat," a genetic expression in the DNA of HIV that it requires to replicate. Other agents with this kind of blocking action include curcumin,[191] a nontoxic, anti-inflammatory compound from the well-known curry spice, turmeric (*Curcuma longa* L.),[192] and topotecan, a semi-synthetic anticancer agent. From animal and human data on their toxicity, these compounds would probably not cause intolerable side-effects.[193]

A subject of less recent intrigue concerns the action of this quinone at interfering with the ability of damaged tumor cells to repair themselves, even after the tumors have been treated with anticancer drugs or radiation. Since 1984, researchers at Harvard University Medical School and Dana-Farber Cancer Institute have found *beta*-lapachone a very useful tool for understanding the mechanisms of tumor cell resistance to treatment.[194] For example, in malignant melanoma cells previously resistant to radiation, *beta*-lapachone, *following* anticancer drugs or low doses of radiation, greatly reduced the ability of these cells to repair their broken strands of DNA, which would otherwise allow them to reestablish themselves. *Beta*-lapachone appears to alter the ability of tumor cells to repair their damaged DNA by activating and modifying the actions of an enzyme (topoisomerase I) that many kinds of tumor cells use for reconnecting broken DNA and thereby replicating.[195]

The alkaloid camptothecin, an anticancer agent derived from a Chinese tree (*Camptothecin acuminata*) used for centuries in herbal formulas to treat cancer, also affects the activity of the enzyme topoisomerase I.[196] Rather than activating and modifying the enzyme as *beta*-lapachone does, however, the alkaloid *inactivates* the enzyme,[197] a feat most anticancer drugs can't perform. There is reason to believe that because of this shortfall, many tumors have shown resistance to many of the chemotherapy agents available. The National Cancer Institute is currently testing a chemically modified form of the alkaloid called topotecan, which has fewer side-effects than the original compound.[198, 199] Since DNA-repair modifiers greatly enhance the anticancer effects of chemotherapy drugs, it is conceivable that the dosages of chemotherapy might be lowered, thereby reducing the risks of side-effects. And if topoisomerase-active agents prove more effective than the arsenal of agents now in use, *beta*-lapachone, probably in combination with other agents,[200] could be next in line for clinical studies.[201]

With the identification of this enzyme system, the search for substances to interfere with tumor cell DNA repair (DNA-repair modifiers) from plants long used to treat cancer in folk medicine may continue to yield promising finds. Already, inhibitors of topoisomerase II activity, which is used by

HIV-1 to replicate, have been isolated from the Cairo morning glory (*Ipomoea cairica*), a tropical shrub from Africa and Asia.[202] But a word of caution must attend the use of herbal medicines as DNA-repair modifiers, for unless they can be shown not to interfere with the DNA repair of normal cells, the possibility of toxic effects on DNA cannot be outruled. Even without *prior* DNA-damaging agents (such as chemotherapy and radiation), *beta*-lapachone alone causes chromosomal damage and breaks DNA strands.[203] Because other chemically related quinones, such as vitamin K_3 (menadione) and some common quinone-based anticancer drugs have the same or similar action on DNA,[204] the wood extract of pau d'arco can scarcely be thought of as a nontoxic herbal product like the bark. Even though the amount of *beta*-lapachone and other quinones in the wood of pau d'arco is small, internal use of the wood extract may be regarded as something more akin to chemotherapy, although undoubtedly much less toxic, while that of the bark may be more akin to immunotherapy, each having some therapeutic features shared by the other.

ACTIVE CONSTITUENTS

Lapachol is a well-known antitumor agent that occurs in the wood. In the bark, lapachol shows up either in minute amounts or not at all.[205, 206] As well as the inner bark itself (*T. heptaphylla* and *T. impetiginosa*), lapachol activated human immune cells (lymphocytes and granulocytes) in low concentrations.[207] Lymphocytes are cells that mediate immunologic responses and are defined according to the immune operations they perform. Most lymphocytes circulating in the bloodstream are T-lymphocytes, often called T-cells. The granulocytes are white blood cells predominantly found in the blood. Like the macrophage, they devour foreign cells and are directly involved in tissue repair and fighting invading bacteria.

Lapachol is barely soluble in water,[208] and when it does occur in the bark, it occurs only in trace amounts.[209–211] However, Dr. Wagner's team found still other quinones in the bark with immunostimulating activity. Although no one knew they were immuno-active at the time, some of them had already been found in a pau d'arco from the Brazilian coast called the *pao de tamanco*, or *tabebuya*, a Tupi-Guarani Indian name meaning "ant wood"; ants were often found inhabiting the hollowed twigs. This was the tree that the entire genus of *Tabebuia* would later be named after.[212, 213] It was also the tree that scientists eventually used to solve the riddle of which, if any, active quinones occurred in the barks of pau d'arco used in South American folk medicine and in commercially available pau d'arco used by North Americans.

Pao de tamanco is a medium or small white-flowered tree (*Tabebuia cassinoides* [Lam.] A.P. Candolle) found in fresh-water swamps along the central coast of Brazil.[214] This tree received its common name from an old Brazilian practice of using its lightweight wood to make wooden shoes (tamancos). The bark contains several antitumor quinones. In 1982 chemists at the Virginia Polytechnic Institute and State University reported they had discovered that an alcoholic extract of the stem-bark held definite antileukemic activity. When they tested the bark for antitumor effects, they found significant activity and discovered three new quinones similar to lapachol yet considerably more active.[215]

The bark of the pao de tamanco is applied in Brazilian folk medicine to increase urination. Records state that "5 grams of new bark should be used per 300 grams of water in order to provide 3 to 5 cups a day." The tea was reported as having "good cleansing effects on the liver and spleen." The fruit peel is also diuretic and when made into a tea was said to contain a "hypnotic" substance.[216] Other folk uses in Brazil include the treatment of anemia and intestinal ailments and the stimulation of appetite.[217]

The same quinones found in the bark of the pao de tamanco occur in the barks of many pau d'arco used in folk medicine.[218–222] These findings have inspired Japanese scientists. Two universities in Kyoto discovered that an alcoholic extract of the inner bark (*T. impetiginosa*) significantly reduced tumor formation resulting from a carcinogen, and in another test, it showed anti–tumor-promoting activity. A water extract was effective, too, only a little less potent.[223]

Other investigators in Japan, including the National Cancer Center Research Institute (Japan's equivalent of the NCI in the United States), recently reported that an extract (alcoholic) of Brazilian pau d'arco bark

(*T. impetiginosa*) showed antitumor activity (against Sarcoma 180 ascites) in mice. In the course of their study, they found the same immunostimulating quinones that Dr. Wagner had uncovered in Munich, and in the test tube the same quinones were active against an experimental leukemia (L1210). Antitumor activity was also found in mice with leukemia (P-388), but the level of activity was not statistically significant.[224] Two of the quinones combined provided a 15 percent increase in lifespan compared to mice not receiving the quinones (100 mg/kg/day for five days).[225] Indeed, the University of Munich had found them to be weakly immunostimulating.[226] One of these, called kigelinone, was previously isolated from the wood of an African tree (*Kigelia pinnata*) related to pau d'arco.[227] In 1994, Professor Shinichi Ueda at Kyoto University reported that he was continuing the research with pau d'arco (*T. impetiginosa*) bark because it holds a wealth of quinones and very "promising therapeutic effects." In one assay, he found that the "cancer preventive" activity of kigelinone was 10,000 times greater than that of lapachol.[228] Because of their possible future potential, furanonaphthoquinones from pau d'arco were patented in Japan in 1988 as "neoplasm inhibitors" and anticancer agents for leukemia.[229]

It was at about the same time that Brazilian scientists discovered that the bark of a pau d'arco (*T. ochracea*), one with tannish colored flowers with yellow throats, contained a quinone with a wide spectrum of activity.[230] In particular, they were encouraged by its action against the parasites that cause a tropical infection (Chaga's disease)[231] and malaria.[232] Another team in Brazil have found pain-relieving action from a wood extract of a yellow pau d'arco (*T. chrysotricha*). They found lapachol was also analgesic, and one of the quinones they isolated was identical to one of the immunostimulating quinones previously found in the inner bark (*T. impetiginosa*).[233]

TURNING TO THE LEAVES

Activity studies of the leaves of pau d'arco have been few and very far between. This is unfortunate, since there is some indication that the leaves may be more potent than the bark, and their harvest, carried out at an ecologically safe level, would be much less traumatic to the trees.

In a 1963 study, the leaves of *T. barbata* showed five times the enhancement of phagocytic activity that the bark of the same tree provided,[234] but since then no one has taken up the study of the immunopotentiating actions of the leaves. In recent times, a group at the Pharmacognosy Department of Assuit University in Egypt have analyzed the leaves of a yellow-flowered pau d'arco[235] (incorrectly identified as *T. pentaphylla* Hemsl.).[236, 237] The leaves were collected when the tree was flowering at the Aswan Botanic Island in Egypt. With the assistance of Dr. Norman R. Farnsworth at the College of Pharmacy at the University of Illinois, Chicago, the researchers isolated a compound called betulinic acid and found that it was active against two kinds of tumor cells (P388 lymphocytic leukemia and KB cells, *in vitro*) highly predictive of antitumor activity in people. They also found the bioflavonoids quercetin and kaempferol.[238]

From their detailed drawings of the various tree parts, there's no question that the Egyptian team had their hands on a *Tabebuia*, but it wasn't the species they thought. Mistaken identity has occurred repeatedly with pau d'arco, and it will probably happen again. The tree studied was likely a hybrid of *T. rosea*, a native of the tropical Americas widely cultivated in India. We took it up in the previous chapter with reports that the Huastec Mayans in Mexico use the bark to treat cancer of the uterus or vagina, malaise, and ulcers and to wash wounds and sores. Herbalists in India use this tree as a diuretic, a fever reducer, a "hypnotic agent," and an antidote for poisoning and infections.[239]

Betulinic acid (a triterpene) occurs in birch trees (*Betula* sp.) and was originally isolated as an antitumor compound from a shrub (*Hyptis emoryi* Torr.) found in the southwest United States.[240] The seeds (*chia*) from this shrub are eaten by the indigenous people of Mexico, and the leaves of related species in Mexico and Central America provide a tea used to treat fevers and stomach ache.[241] The same applications are found in the Peruvian Amazon with *Hyptis* species found there,[242] and in Brazil the leaf tea of salva-de marajó (*H. incana* Briq.) is taken for stomach ache and the leaf juice used as a topical treatment for sunburn.[243]

In addition to the early finding of antitumor activity, betulinic acid has shown inflammation-inhibiting and tumor-preventive activity. When two mg of betulinic acid was applied to the ears of mice, the action of a powerful inflammatory chemical was inhibited by 87 percent.[244] A similar compound in the leaves of pau d'arco called betulin[245] inhibited inflammation by 94 percent.[246] In future, it may be useful to find herbal medicines that contain these compounds for possible applications against inflammatory conditions. The wild iris (*Iris missouriensis* Nutt.), which was widely used by Indians in the western United States to treat toothache,[247] and the leaves of *fukanoki* (*Schefflera octophylla*), still used by Vietnamese and Chinese herbalists specifically as an anti-inflammatory, both contain betulinic acid.[248, 249] Betulin is abundant in the outer bark and leaves of the European birch (*Betula alba* L.).[250]

Skin tumors topically induced by a chemical (DMBA) plus an inflammatory agent applied two times a week were found in 100 percent of mice, with 21.1 tumors each. But if betulinic acid was applied prior to the chemicals, tumor incidence was only 8.8 per mouse. That's a 60 percent reduction in tumor incidence. At the Department of Pharmacy at Nihon University in Chiba, Japan, the authors of that study concluded that since compounds of these types (sterols and triterpenes) are found throughout the kingdom of edible plants, they may be of considerable importance for the prevention of cancer.[251] To that one would have to add medicinal plants, which continue to occupy researchers as the main source for finding these compounds in medicinally active forms.[252–255]

Still other inflammation-preventive substances occurring in the leaves include *alpha*-amyrin, which is also found in the bark, and oleanolic acid.[256] These showed inflammation inhibition rates of 86 and 73 percent, respectively.[257]

Originally found in olive leaves, oleanolic acid is a triterpene with tumor-inhibiting activity of interest to the Japanese Ministry of Health and Welfare for the "chemoprevention" of cancer through the diet. Since 1983 in Japan, isolating and identifying nontoxic tumor-inhibitors that occur in plants has been part of a strategy to delay cancer onset and, ideally, to inhibit the initiation of tumor development or *carcinogenesis*. Vitamins C and E, *beta*-carotene, and other natural tumor inhibitors found in the plants we eat are being tested in eighteen long-term human trials to see which supplements best interfere with cancer development. Oleanolic acid, which is experimentally effective against skin cancers, is one of the most recent prospects for inclusion in these trials.[258]

The search for cancer-preventive substances in the plant kingdom now extends to India, where oleanolic acid derived from flowers of the Java plum (*Eugenia jambolana* Lam.) showed excellent antioxidant activity in liver cells from rats. As a pre-treatment, oleanolic acid provided a potent 90 percent protection from liver damage caused by free radicals oxidizing fatty cells. Even as a post-treatment, free radical damage to the liver cells was reversed with oleanolic acid by 25 percent.[259]

Tissue damage to the heart and liver by chemotherapy is a major threat to the survival of cancer patients. For many years, patients receiving chemotherapy in the West have been forbidden to take antioxidant supplements such as vitamin C or E while undergoing therapy for fear that they would diminish the cell-killing action of the drugs. But now, that fear is starting to fade and researchers are actively seeking antioxidants with the goal of applying them against cancer. Toward this aim, researchers in India have been experimenting with oleanolic acid and have found it to be a "strong protector." In the laboratory, damage to heart and liver cells caused by the free radicals produced from the quinone anticancer drug adriamycin was inhibited by 21 percent in heart cells and by 49 percent in liver cells.[260]

In the United States, other investigators have discovered that as a pre-treatment oleanolic acid can protect mice from liver damage caused by the heavy metal cadmium.[261] In China, oleanolic acid has already been applied in humans as a nontoxic treatment for hepatitis,[262] and there are indications that it may also be useful in the treatment of arthritis. In a battery of tests in mice, oleanolic acid taken orally was at least comparable in potency to aspirin (acetyl salicylic acid), but it doesn't operate by the same mechanisms.[263]

Also found in the bark,[264] oleanolic acid is of considerable interest to the development of "differentiation-inducing" agents, substances that cause leukemia cells to transform into cells with characteristics of immune cells, such as cell-gobbling (phagocytic), motility and enzymatic actions.[265] As early as 1977, leukemia cells from a patient with acute promyelocytic leukemia were differentiated into macrophages and granulocytes by a group of American immunologists at the National Cancer Institute.[266] As bizarre as this may seem, differentiation-inducers are now "expected" to become a new class of anticancer drugs for the simple reason that they can induce cancerous cells "to differentiate into normal cells." Derived from an extract of clove buds (*Syzgium aromaticum* Merril and Perry), oleanolic acid showed such "potent" activity in differentiating myeloid leukemia cells from mice into macrophage-like cells that in 1992, Dr. Kaoru Umehara and team at the University of Shizuoka in Japan described the action as "remarkable."[267] A year later, they reported that they had found several other compounds with this activity in the fruits of burdock (*Arctium lappa* L.),[268] another very common herb. Before moving on, it is important to note that some bioflavonoids have this action, too.[269] Kaempferol, which was also found in the leaves of *Tabebuia*,[270] is one of the most highly active.[271]

UNDISSOLVED MYSTERIES

Tests show that most of the pau d'arco barks sold in North America hold immuno-active quinones.[272] But it turns out that these aren't the only substances in the bark that have the distinction of boosting the immune system.

The most complete breakdown of pau d'arco (*T. impetiginosa*, northwest Argentina) to date was performed by Bernhard Kreher, Ph.D., at the Institute of Pharmaceutical Biology, University of Munich. Along with such familiar compounds as salicylic acid (4-hydroxybenzoic acid), vanillin, vanillic acid (4-hydroxy-3-methoxybenzoic acid), and anisic acid (4-methoxybenzoic acid),[273] a topical anti-inflammatory[274] and tyrosinase-inhibiting[275] compound also found in anise (*Pimpinella anisum* L.), he found a total of seven substances with immunostimulating action. Five were quinones and two were something no one had expected. The most abundant of these (about one mg/gram of bark) was a type of benzoic acid called veratric acid (3,4-dimethoxybenzoic acid).[276] The other, verataldehyde, was only weakly active at stimulating the cell-gobbling activity of granulocytes; however, at stimulating the proliferation of lymphocytes, this substance was very active. Kreher found a 66.2 percent increase in proliferation from 100 nanograms (billionths of a gram) per milliliter of cells.[277] Unfortunately, verataldehyde oxidizes to veratric acid upon exposure to light.[278]

Veratric acid, a by-product of lignin decomposition in wood,[279] is also the major inactive metabolite of mebeverine, a smooth-muscle relaxant used as an antispasmodic in irritable bowel syndrome and duodenal ulcers.[280–282] But apart from Dr. Kreher's finding of an immunostimulating action,[283] it has no other known activity.[284–286] Veratric acid stimulated the proliferation of lymphocytes by 27.3 percent (ten nanograms/ml) and the phagocytic activity of granulocytes by 32.2 percent (one nanogram/ml). Dr. Kreher writes that veratric acid and verataldehyde were identified as "good immune stimulators."[287]

Finally, the question remains as to what compounds are going to be found from analyzing the bark available in the marketplace. Attempting to answer that question with respect to quinones, two independent groups have examined pau d'arco.[288,289] Only one group, a Canadian team headed by Dennis V.C. Awang, Ph.D., then at the Bureau of Drug Research of Health Canada in Ottawa, detected the presence of lapachol, and then only in minute amounts in two out of twelve samples of bark that he prepared as solvent extracts. These amounts were 0.0003 percent and less than 0.00004 percent lapachol. Dr. Awang's group established the presence of quinones related to lapachol in ten pau d'arco products sold in Canada in the usual form of loose bark for tea. Although Dr. Awang was not able to establish their respective quantities, their amounts were apparently minute. No quinones were detected in three commercial alcoholic extracts of the bark.[290]

In 1992 a British team headed by P.J. Houghton, Ph.D., at the Chelsea Department of Pharmacy of King's College of London, found quinones to be absent in a single commercial sample of pau d'arco identified as *Tabebuia impetiginosa*. Dr. Houghton explained that activity studies of the bark to date have usually been performed using solvents not found in commercial extracts and homemade teas of pau d'arco, and for that reason he endeavored to examine the "tea" for quinones. After purchasing pau d'arco from a London shop, he boiled the bark and then concentrated the liquid by freeze-drying. He did not detect any lapachol or any related quinones in this concentrate. However, he did find the presence of four major compounds in the tea, two of which he identified as triterpenoids and phenolics, but the exact identities and activities of these have yet to be determined.[291] These same kinds of compounds have been detected in a simple water extract of pau d'arco bark from northeast Argentina (*Tabebuia heptaphylla*), which also appeared to be devoid of quinones,[292] and the trunk bark of a yellow pau d'arco, *T. serratifolia*.[293] Triterpenoids of many types and actions occur in the plants of the tropical Americas,[294] and it will be most interesting to learn what turns up in teas and alcoholic extracts of pau d'arco.

Dr. Houghton's findings reminded me of a letter I received years earlier from Dr. Kreher concerning the identity of active constituents in the tea and my curiosity about the presence of poorly soluble quinones. He pointed out that although the solubility of lapachol in water is very small, the amounts required for immunostimulation were remarkably small and one could not outrule the possibility of greater solubility of lapachol and related quinones in traditional preparations (crude extracts) where the quinones may occur in emulsion with "other compounds, i.e. triterpenes."[295]

As their name implies, terpenes take their name from the "turp" in turpentine oil, the source of the terpenoids known as pinenes. Besides oleanolic acid, other well-known terpenoids include the monoterpenes menthol, thymol, citronellal, camphor, limonene from pine needle oil, the expectorant cineol from eucalyptus oil, and the antitumor agent taxol (a diterpene) from the yew tree (*Taxus brevifolia*). Triterpenes occur in plants as saponins, steroids, and sterols.[296] In these classes some of the better-known medicinally active triterpenes occur in licorice root, gingko leaves, Siberian ginseng, and the reishi mushroom.[297, 298]

Dr. Hildebert Wagner had found that a water extract of the inner bark (*T. impetiginosa*) enhanced phagocytic activity of immune cells by 40 percent from only fifty micrograms of extract/ml of cells.[299] And Dr. Kreher found a strong (48.8 percent) increase of this activity in granulocytes from only twenty-five nanoliters (billionths of a liter!) of the water extract. As for quinones from the bark, two are noteworthy, kigelinone and 8-hydroxy-2-(1'-hydroxyethyl)furanonaphthoquinone, identical except for the first number. Combined (100 to the minus 15th or femtograms/ml), they produced a 23.8 percent stimulation of granulocytic cell-gobbling activity, and a higher dose of ten nanograms (billionths of a gram) stimulated lymphocytic proliferation by 40.8 percent.[300] From these extremely low concentrations, I have to wonder again about the people with yeast syndrome who took their pau d'arco tea diluted—a drop or two of tea per liter of water—and yet claimed they found benefits.[301]

Is it possible that quinones were found to be absent in the bark teas because the amounts were too small to show up in the test systems used and that these amounts *are* causing immunostimulation? Some authorities discount this model outright, while others believe it to be entirely plausible.

One kind of compound found in both the extract (alcoholic) and the tea (water extract) of the inner bark (*T. impetiginosa*) is saponins, the substances that generally cause herbal teas to foam when shaken.[302] Saponins with antitumor activity, however weak (27.8 percent tumor growth inhibition of Sarcoma 180 in mice), have been isolated from the inner bark of Brazilian pau d'arco (*T. impetiginosa*) by Japanese scientists who then patented them as antitumor agents.[303] High amounts (3 to 4 percent) of saponins have been found in the wood of *T. impetiginosa* and *T. heptaphylla*[304] and moderate amounts were detected in the water and alcoholic extracts of inner barks of these species in Brazil.[305, 306] These saponins appear to be of the steroidal type.[307] As noted earlier, saponins can increase the availability of other active constituents in medicinal plant preparations by increasing their solubility in water and by enhancing their digestive tract absorption.[308]

As the mysteries of pau d'arco's active constituents continue to unfold, we may take solace in the fact that once these are established, quality can be monitored to provide us with the best of barks. In the meantime, let us not forget that this is a good-tasting tea enjoyed daily by millions of people in Brazil, Portugal, Japan, North America, and other parts of the world, many of whom prefer its taste over that of other teas.

The need for new immunomodulators may be more fruitfully met through a continued appraisal of traditional medical systems than by an attempt to design our own. The relative safety of traditional medicines by virtue of centuries of use may be known only empirically, but owing to a long history of use, focusing on medicinal plants will save the time and considerable expense of a completely random trek through the plant kingdom. The added possibility of finding properties uncharted by folklore or pharmacology offers incentives both for underdeveloped nations—in desperate need of inexpensive and readily available medicines—and for those who would seek to improve medicine in the developed world.

How to lessen the incidence of disease in large populations will continue to be a subject of concerted efforts by entomologists, virologists, pharmacologists, nutritionists, botanists, and anthropologists alike. And while I don't believe herbalism alone is adequate to combat the diversity of diseases the world is facing, I think it conceivable that through the judicious use of medicinal plants, large populations will be able to achieve a generally enhanced resistance, or what is known as the *immunoprophylaxis* of disease. Meeting such a demand represents one of the greatest challenges of medicine for this century and the next.

Pau d'arco's potential in this task will become clarified only as interest in herbal immunostimulants continues to grow. At the same time, this area should not overshadow the possibility of utilizing pau d'arco in research aimed at treatments for any one of the medical problems indicated by folk uses attending this plant.

LOOKING FOR TOXICITY

During the 1960s, one concern raised repeatedly in Brazil was the very practical aspect of safety.[309-311] After all, the masses were drinking *snake oil* that no one of medical authority was really sure about. The same concern has naturally been raised in North America.[312, 313]

At conferences and seminars to determine the merit of pau d'arco, Brazilian authorities referred to the works of Dr. Frederick W. Freise,[314] a chemist who had undertaken the fascinating and tedious chore of recording folk-medicinal uses of Brazilian plants during the first half of this century. From his writings it appears that not all pau d'arco are safe to use as teas.

Noting side-effects from the bark of certain pau d'arco, as well as from their wood, Dr. Freise's reports include some nasty reactions to a yellow pau d'arco,[315] *T. umbellata* (Sonder) Sandw.[316] These resulted from infusions (teas) of the bark and, even more pronounced, from the wood. He found the tea caused abnormal swellings like burns and "skin pustules" to form. The throat became affected with skin loss and "bloody wounds." Dr. Freise wrote, "Because of this, the [alcoholic extract] of the drug should be avoided."[317] For those who would use this pau d'arco, he recommended caution. If the tea was made any stronger than one part bark to ten parts water, the user would experience "painful vomiting accompanied with blood and parts of the intestinal mucous." Much the same precaution was given for another yellow-flowered pau d'arco, *T. pedicellata*, in Brazil,[318] while in Paraguay the yellow-flowered *paratodo* (*T. argentea*,[319] now correctly identified as *T. aurea*[320]) is part of a formula used by indigenous people to induce abortion (with ruta (*Ruta graveolens*) and caroa (*Jacaranda mimosifolia*).[321] One might also inquire as to why the Tikuna Indians of Colombia take the bark decoction of the yellow-flowered *hua-ri* (*Tabebuia neochrysantha* A. Gentry) in a dose of only "an eighth of a cup" three times daily to treat chronic anemia, malaria, and the pain of an ulcer.[322] Unwanted side-effects from a larger dose than this is a plausible explanation.[323]

Obviously, one cannot use just any pau d'arco. According to several of my informants, the bark of a yellow pau d'arco has already been sold in the United States, and in at least one case the reactions were as Dr. Freise forewarned. But what species and whether the bark was in fact a pau d'arco remain unknown. It is doubtful that *all* yellow pau d'arco are toxic. The inner bark of *T. serratifolia*, for example, provided no toxic effects in mice given 1,000 mg of the extract (90 percent ethanol) per kilo of body weight, or 100 mg/kg intravenously.[324]

Dr. Freise designated the inner bark of a purple pau d'arco (*T. impetiginosa*), along with the yellow species given, as providing teas "used as an astringent in gargling in cases of [inflammation of the mucous membrane of the mouth] or throat wounds, mainly in ulcers caused by syphilis." Although he made no mention of side-effects from the bark of any species other than the yellow and tannish examples noted, it appears that some species have the opposite effect, having been found instead to remedy an inflamed throat or mouth.[325]

Further to the safety of purple pau d'arco, Professor Valter Accorsi writes that in 1967 the Ministry of Health for the State of São Paulo "proved" there was no toxicity.[326] Teodoro Meyer's statements on the safety of his bark "elixir" were more explicit:

It may be taken in massive doses without fear and it may be combined with other medication, no matter how active the latter is; and it is as suitable for children as it is for adults. It helps to reduce counter-reactions to medications in general and specifically to antibiotics, thus allowing other medications to work more effectively and reducing the danger of toxic effect upon the liver.[327]

Meyer added that neither was there a problem of toxicity with the individual barks used in his extract.[328] Although a decoction of *T. heptaphylla* from northeast Argentina is "recommended in folk medicine for inducing abortion,"[329] I have seen no evidence for the effectiveness of this and expect that other plants in a formula that merely happened to include the bark are the real abortive plants.[330] Finally, Professor Accorsi provides the following observations regarding alcoholic extracts of pau d'arco:

Many people who use too much of the extract (of the inner bark) . . . in the day, will feel a slight irritation, a sort of itchiness, although it is of no consequence. With a lessening of doses everything goes back to normal. I think that in these cases the people took too much of the extract than they were supposed to. Only this, and I repeat that this does not present any inconvenience . . . a person can take five grams of extract per kilogram of body weight, daily, with no damage.[331]

Meyer's advice to allow the hot tea to cool before drinking[332] may be advisable for any frequently consumed tea rich in catechin tannins not taken with milk to bind the tannins; even if only from long-term, excessive intake of plants high in catechins, the combination of hot liquid with those tannins has been associated with tissue damage leading to cancer of the esophagus.[333] Such a precaution may not apply to all pau d'arco teas, for in many areas of Brazil they appear to have only small amounts of tannin.[334]

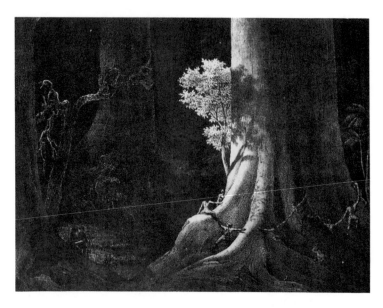

Botanists in the Amazonian forest of 1840–1906. From Carlos F. P. De Martius and Augustus G. Eichler, *Flora Brasiliensis, 1840–1906,* vol. 1, part 1 (Weinheim, Germany: Verlag von J. Cramer, 1965), reprint.

FIVE

Thieves in the Forest

As early as the 1950s in Argentina, it was obvious to Teodoro Meyer that with continued economic expansionism South America's trees were facing perilous consequences.[1] Attempting to curtail the inevitable, he established the Friends of the Trees Society, "to prevent the unnecessary and irrational destruction of vegetation."[2]

Losing miles of our tropical rain forests is a gloomy prospect, one for which we are told the consequences promise a significant loss of planetary oxygen and the alteration of global weather patterns for all time. The Amazonian rain forest provides almost 50 percent of the world's supply of regenerated air. The rain forests of this region alone are therefore vital to the survival of humankind.

While we may be grateful that this much information makes the news, too little attention is being paid to the peril facing tropical herbs. Even as I write, medicines are being lost forever and with them an ancient cultural resource that stands to save us untold years of investigation: Without the native herbalists and their shamans to guide us, how will we know which plants, out of the hundreds of thousands of species available, to spend precious time in studying?

The Amazon holds about two-thirds of the entire tropical rain forest of the world. There, the rate of slaughter is feverish. At five acres an hour,[3] it poses a threat to all humankind. Already one-fifth of the Amazonian forest lies in waste. Map to map, that's a chunk of land exceeding the entire area of the Yukon.[4] In the Brazilian Amazon alone, from 1978 to 1989 deforestation averaged 2.1 million hectares a year.[5] Just how many medicines are now lost is impossible to calculate, for several or more medicines can originate in a single species. In Brazil, where there are about 120,000 native plant species, the chemical constituents of over 99 percent remain unknown.[6] One can only guess at the number of useful herbs and medicines awaiting discovery (or rediscovery) and their potential impact on the world economy in this one tropical region. Harvard University ethnobotanist Richard Evans Schultes reminds us of some Amazonian plants already of major economic impact that we tend to take for granted. Among them he gives the pineapple (*Ananas comosus* [L.] Merrill), tapioca (*Manihot esculenta* Crantz), and cacao (*Theobroma cacao* L.) for making chocolate. He notes that the Aztecs flavored their *chocolatl* preparations with the vanilla bean (*Vanilla planifolia*), and from the bark of *achiotl* they added the orange-yellow dye known as achiote (*Bixa orellana* L.), a dye rich in vitamin A which finds use today in Western industrialized countries for coloring cheese, margarine, soups, soaps, cosmetics, and paints. Achiote was long used as a body paint by numerous tribes in South America. Rubber, coca, the Brazil nut, and a seemingly endless number of ornamental plants should scarcely need mentioning.[7]

PERILS OF PAU D'ARCO

By 1988 sales of pau d'arco had reached the $200 million mark.[8] Most of the pau d'arco available is from trees that are first cut down for their valuable wood, there being no point in letting it go to waste at the mills. Although an alternative method of harvesting the bark without harming the trees is a well-known native practice (see chapter 3), it doesn't provide the amount of bark commerce usually insists on and is much slower than cutting down the trees first. A pau d'arco tree reaches maturity in twenty years in Brazil, but it will be sufficiently grown for harvesting after only eight years.

Cultivation of herbs was encouraged at a meeting of the World Health Organization in Rome in 1979, when Dr. A. Bonati emphasized the importance of herb cultivation to our future. The practice, he stated, "represents the most simple solution of a problem which will become more and more serious: the increasing consumptions of certain medicinal plants which cannot be supplied by plants in their wild state, not to mention the ecological problems."[9]

Obviously, there is a great need for cultivation that goes beyond even matters of ecology and supply. Factors in the field altering the quality of an herb or its yield are matters routinely encountered by producers of medicinal plants. To provide consistent quality, cultivation of many plants in one area facilitates monitoring of active compounds, once these become known.

More than one writer today has found the decimation of the rain forest advancing so fast that the species in its path are gone before there's time to so much as tell about them. Shortly before completing this book, I learned that we now face the prospect of losing tahuari, a pau d'arco the shamans in Peru regard very highly. In 1987, following one of his regular visits to Peru, the late Dr. Alwyn H. Gentry, curator at the Missouri Botanical Garden in St. Louis and the world authority on the botany of *Tabebuia*, reported that tahuari had been all but exhausted. Undaunted and unscrupulous, harvesters are now substituting for tahuari (*Tabebuia serratifolia*, *T. incana*, and other *Tabebuia* in this region) the similar-textured bark of a completely unrelated tree (*Cariniana* sp.).[10,11] The more knowledgeable herbalists and older ones who once gathered the genuine bark all spoke of the *Cariniana*, the "false tahuari."[12] In the street-markets of Iquitos, *Cariniana* bark is being sold for the same uses people made of the real tahuari, such as curing diabetes, cancer, and an assortment of other conditions. But today *Cariniana* is facing decimation, too! Around Iquitos the false tahuari has also become scarce. Gentry found the few survivors remaining were bare-trunked past the height of a man and girdled with structures erected to reap more bark.[13]

ENDANGERED PAU D'ARCO[14]

Tabebuia rosea	Highly sought in Central America, Mexico, Panama, and northwest South America
T. angustata	Among the top timbers logged in West Indies

T. heterophylla	Among the top timbers logged in West Indies
T. billbergii	Among most important woods logged in Ecuador
T. chrysantha	Among most important woods logged in Ecuador
T. insignis	Main native tree added to pulp at the Jari plant in Brazil
T. guayacan	Now wanted by U.S. importers
T. heptaphylla	Prized in south Brazil and Paraguay; most good timber now gone in south Brazil; most important species of trees logged in east Paraguay; being logged as the first choice timber at Río Jejui-Mí, Paraguay, where the forests were otherwise still "intact"; Paraná Forest in Paraguay now main source for all *Tabebuia* in region.

The disappearance of trees in Peru is especially painful. The upper regions of the Amazon in that country contain a greater diversity of trees than any other region on the planet. Gentry's surveys, published in the January 1988 issue of the *Proceedings of the National Academy of Sciences,* show they reach 300 species per hectare—more than the record previously held by Southeast Asia by as much as 200 species! Even so, diversity and density are two different things. Because plants exist *interdependently*, when one species goes, others are bound to follow.

During one of his treks to the Choco region of Columbia, where he was accompanied by *National Geographic* (see issue of January 1983), Gentry deplored a loss of species we can never retrieve. With the removal of the larger trees (and, believe it or not, some of *those* have yet to be studied), overnight we are losing species that they have been sheltering for thousands of years.[15] Further compounding these losses, the majority remain so much a mystery they may as well be legends.

In the same region, less than a square mile of rain forest shelters 1,000 species of plants. When we stop to consider that in all of Britain the number of shrubs, trees, and herbaceous plants amounts to but 1,450 species, Gentry's call for urgent action resounds with a warning not only for us, but also for generations to come. Never mind their potential in medicine or as subjects for writers, the rain forest plants are becoming extinct even before we have a chance to catalog them.[16]

In August 1993, Dr. Gentry died in a plane crash while surveying uncharted forests of Ecuador. He is sorely missed. His collection of some 70,000 plant specimens in the tropical Americas exceeded that of any other botanist alive today. What he knew about the botany of woody plants in the tropics was unmatched. Dr. Peter H. Raven, director of the Missouri Botanical Garden, where Gentry worked, regarded him as more knowledgeable about Latin American plants than any other person in the entire world.[17]

VANISHING SHAMANS

One authority after another has returned from the forests to repeat a different kind of warning: shamanism is dying, and fast. At the New York Botanical Garden, Michael Balick tells us that young people no longer value the knowledge of the shaman, and so vast repositories of herbal knowledge are going to the grave.[18] After many years in the forests of the Amazon investigating the plant uses of indigenous peoples, ethnobotanist E. Wade Davis, Ph.D., has become an outspoken witness to the current erosion of shamanism and a proponent of the need to preserve that knowledge before all is lost. Author of *The Serpent and the Rainbow* (Simon and Schuster, 1986), Davis hopes that the movie titled after his book, about the recovery of a "zombie" formula from Haiti that may prove valuable to medical research, will entice the young and wealthy of Wall Street to pursue the riches of the *real* jungle—while they still can. It was Davis who reported a pau d'arco being regularly used everywhere in the Amazon as a treatment for cancer, "by both folk and western doctors."[19]

During his studies of ayahuasquero, Dr. Luis Luna found that in Peru the message is the same. Don Sergio, another of the shamans he interviewed, was forty-two at the time.[20] He was the youngest *vegetalista* (one who acquires medical knowledge from plant spirits) Luna had encountered. Sergio related that the spirits of the Amazon are not pleased. The noise from an advancing technology, broadcast by drills, motorcycles, and cars, is disturbing their world. In all his years studying the healing tradition in Peru, Dr. Luna found not a single shaman attended by a successor. The young are increasingly turning to the things of civilization, be they transistor radios, watches, motorcycles, leather boots, or peer pressure to consume alcohol, "the drug of the colonists."[21]

Everywhere in the Peruvian Amazon, cultures are being leveled as the economy erodes: capital reinvestment is practically nil, and everything is becoming costly, while wages stay low. Like the vagrant farmers in Brazil, who out of poverty and ignorance destroy one patch of forest, plant their crops, deplete the soil, and then go somewhere else and burn again, the population is highly transient, following a demand for a product, exhausting it, and then moving on.[22] In 1986, Luna lamented the inevitable:

> The demographic pressure on the Amazon is causing great changes. 5.7% of the forest of the Peruvian Amazon has been destroyed, and the prognosis is that by the year 2000, 15.2% of the jungle [12 million hectares] will have been cleared out, with unimaginable climatic, ecological and social consequences.[23]

In order to rescue herbal traditions, action must be taken on a local level to integrate the new medicine with the old.[24] As one who knows the real value of this approach, to both public health and the advancement of medical knowledge, Dr. Elaine Elizabetsky of the Federal University of Pará in Belém, Brazil, writes that it is not only possible, but also "necessary to improve the interaction between folk and modern medical systems." Furthermore, she adds, there need not be "conflict between indigenous curers and their biomedical counterparts," as evidenced by the integration already found in Malaysia, China, India, and Brazil.[25] But then Brazil is easily the third largest domestic herb market in the world.

In *Healers of the Andes* (University of Utah Press, 1987), author Joseph Bastien has documented what appears to be such an integration in Bolivia. There an herbal revival is now clearly recognizable. The key factor is that Kallawayas and Western doctors are beginning to work together. In the hopeful event that an alliance continues, Bolivia may find an affordable and effective means of health care while simultaneously preserving a tradition of international acclaim. The educational and promotional efforts of the Kallawaya, combined with the willingness of Bolivia's physicians to acknowledge that not all is known to Western medicine, may well serve to provide models for the preservation and integration of herbalism in neighboring countries.[26, 27]

In any one of these rapidly changing regions, such an integration requires tremendous care and, of course, expert attention.[28] Conceivably, the integration of folk and Western medicine could begin on its own. As physicians become more knowledgeable of plant medicines and witness the medical consequences of economic pressures, I believe a natural integration is inevitable. For example, the 150,000 inhabitants of Iquitos are served by a regional hospital where, although treatments are Western, physicians encourage patients to go on using herbs. Doctors in Iquitos figure about 70 percent of the local population do just that. Nevertheless, there are clear signs that the old practice is dying.[29]

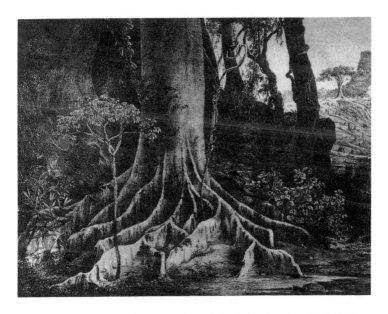

A slash and burn in the former province of Rio de Janeiro, circa 1840–1906. From Carlos F. P. De Martius and Augustus G. Eichler, *Flora Brasiliensis, 1840–1906,* vol. 1, part 1 (Weinheim, Germany: Verlag von J. Cramer, 1965), reprint.

Nicole Maxwell is a research associate of the New York Museum of the American Indian and a fellow of the Royal Geographic Society of London. Now in her eighties, she spent most of the last thirty years living among the natives of the Amazon and has cataloged hundreds of their medicinal plants.[30] Maxwell attests to the efficacy of traditional medicine after being cured herself. She writes that by taking a crude extract of the root bark off a big shrub known as *hiporuru* (a member of the Euphorbiaceae family), like others before her she became free from osteoarthritis,[31] a noninflammatory but painful degenerative disease of the joints. Today the loss of such prescriptions is what concerns her most. Maxwell warns that it is not only that the variety of plants is no longer what it was, but also that the young people would rather take medicines that come in packages. Owing to the encroaching development of the Amazon and because the herbal teachings are completely oral, she predicts that in two or more decades no one will be knowledgeable of the old cures.[32]

REMEDIES IN THE RAIN

The decimation of our rain forests heralds the loss of potentially billions of dollars in the future discovery and development of new and safer compounds from plant sources—either long used in crude form or still completely unknown. Naturally, the majority would rather avoid drugs altogether. Given a choice, however, today most would opt for a natural product over a synthetic one.

For the year 1980, in the United States alone plant-derived prescriptions reached an estimated consumer cost of eight billion dollars.[33, 34] Half of the plants used originated in the tropics.[35] When one considers that in the same year only forty-one species provided approximately one hundred "useful drugs"—all derived from higher (flowering) plants[36]—and that at most 5 percent of the planet's conservatively estimated 250,000 species have been checked in some way for active compounds,[37] not to explore traditional medicines and to rely largely on synthetics seems an incredible waste.

Maxwell is certain that at a minimum, 30 medicinal plants from her collection of over 600 have modes of action that modern Western medicine would find completely novel. Richard Evans Schultes of Harvard Botanical Museum, the world's most outstanding ethnobotanist, lived among the shamans of the Amazon for thirteen years. The booty of his sojourn is a collection of 24,000 plants. If he's right, 5,000 hold properties that will eventually contribute to the well-being of humankind.[38]

Presently, 7,000 compounds are employed by modern medicine that were originally found in natural products. In their crudest forms, the majority were applied for hundreds of years by healers in Asia, the Americas, and Europe.[39] Common sense would tell us that by taking heed of folk medicine the chances of failure in locating active plants are going to be significantly reduced.[40-42]

Apart from the possibility of rescuing herbs of medicinal value to the industrialized world, imagine their importance to the people in whose own back yards they grow, but who sometimes do not know that such and such a plant would alleviate a particular malady, or that one would work better than another. For developing countries, where populations are undergoing a dramatic increase, herbal research is of inestimable value, for "wild" medicines are often of immediate importance to survival. In some countries, medicinal plants comprise 90 percent of all therapeutic means available.[43] When one considers that, for example, in all of black Africa there are fewer medical doctors than in the metropolitan area of Washington, D.C.,[44] it is clear that the medical needs of the third world will be largely reliant upon herbs and other traditional medicaments for a long time to come. Since a meeting of the World Health Organization in 1977, the fact that herbs are more critical to the survival of humankind than was previously supposed in the industrialized world has gained much wider recognition. The conclusion reached was that perhaps "the most cogent reason for the radical development and promotion of traditional medicine is that it is one of the surest means to achieve total health care coverage of the world population, using acceptable, safe, and economically feasible methods."[45] No matter how we approach it, health care for an entire nation doesn't come cheap. In hospitals alone, Americans are now spending over a million dollars every three minutes, and costs are not coming down.[46]

While massive populations already deplete what little foreign currency the developing countries manage, the cost of importing pharmaceuticals now ranks among the most rapidly draining.[47] Despite considerable per capita expenditures on drugs in developing countries, even by the poorest (from 1982 to 1984 Brazil spent $8.39 per person), the World Health Organization warns the rest of the world that this isn't nearly adequate for their needs.[48] Add to that the current disappearance of plant species—one every day—along with those knowledgeable of their uses, and we can begin to think in terms of losing considerably more than greenery.

But there are still more reasons to protect and better manage the forests of the tropics. As valuable as they may be, pharmaceuticals or primary compounds for their development represent only one facet of an abundance in natural products generously manufactured by the plants of this region. Among the treasures we take so much for granted are such simple things as dyes, gums, oils, waxes, flavors, and fragrances.[49] Add to that the burgeoning market for herbal teas and extracts in North America,[50] which will predictably bring an increasing number of products from the forests of the tropics. In the long run, this will owe not so much to their exotic nature as to the density and diversification of tropical species, automatically raising the number of useful herbs available. But if herbal interests only go to make profits in the short term, they will repeat the crime of their contemporaries—taking what they will and leaving behind a forest of little return.

Endnotes

CHAPTER ONE

1. Julio Bartolo, "*Ervas Medicinais* a Saude Esta Nas Plantas," *Manchete* (Rio de Janeiro), October 2, 1982, 111–15. Translation.
2. Valter Accorsi, University of São Paulo; personal communication, May 1983.
3. Stephany Grozdea, A.S. Grozdea, Ltda., Rio de Janeiro; personal communication, June 1983.
4. Alwyn H. Gentry, Missouri Botanical Garden; personal communication, February 1984.
5. Jônio de Freitas Mota and Manoel Motta, "Casos Positivos Comprovam: Descoberta a Cura do Câncer," *O'Cruzeiro* (São Paulo), March 18, 1967. Translation.
6. Ibid.
7. Ibid.
8. See note 1 above.
9. See note 5 above.
10. Ibid.
11. Ibid.
12. Ibid.
13. Ibid.
14. John G. Fuller, *Arigo: Surgeon of the Rusty Knife* (New York: Thomas Y. Crowell Company, 1974).
15. See note 1 above.
16. Ibid.
17. Ibid.
18. Ibid.
19. Jônio de Freitas Mota and Manoel Motta, "A Conspiraçao do Silêncio," *O'Cruzeiro* (São Paulo), March 25, 1967. Translation.
20. See note 4 above.
21. See note 19 above.
22. See note 4 above.
23. See note 19 above.
24. Fadlo Fraige Filho, São Paulo; personal communication, June 1984.
25. See note 19 above.
26. Ibid.
27. Ibid.
28. Ursula Grüne, "Sobre o Princípio Antidiabético da Pedra-hume-caá, *Myrcia multiflora* (Lam.) D.C." (master's thesis, Federal University of Rio de Janeiro, 1979), 7, citing N. A. Pereira and C. H. Lima, personal communication, 1976.

29. Jônio de Freitas Mota and Manoel Motta, "A Verdade Sobre O ipé-Roxo," *O'Cruzeiro* (São Paulo), June 10, 1967, 10–13.
30. Ibid.
31. Ibid.
32. Ibid.
33. Fadlo Fraige Filho, São Paulo; letter to the author, August 14, 1983.
34. "Cancer: se cura con te¿," *Ultima Linea* (San Miguel de Tucuman, Argentina) 1, no. 12 (October 1967): 10–12. Translation.
35. Teodoro Luis Meyer, Jr., San Miguel de Tucuman, Argentina; letter to the author, February 12, 1984.
36. See note 34 above.
37. F. Spencer et al., "Survey of Plants for Antimalarial Activity," *Lloydia* 10 (1947): 145–74.
38. See note 35 above.
39. Carlos Landa, National University of Tucuman, Argentina; letter to the author, April 13, 1983.
40. Teodoro Meyer, Curriculum Vitae.
41. Teodoro Meyer, "Nuestro aporte: Elixir Lapachol Meyer," San Miguel de Tucuman, Argentina, July 1971. Brochure. Translation. See also notes 34 and 35 above.
42. See note 34 above.
43. T. Meyer, "Arbols Nuevos O Notables del Noroeste Argentino," *Lilloa* 33 (1968): 12–13.
44. See note 35 above.
45. Milan Dimitri and Jose Biloni, *El Libro Del Arbol* (Buenos Aires: Celulosa Argentina, 1973). See also note 41 above. The common name for *Tabebuia* trees in Argentina, "lapacho," is one often found in the marketplace of North America and Europe. The word appears to derive from *lapachar*, meaning a boggy or extremely humid land. However, *lapa* is a Quechua Indian word meaning a gourd or clay jug—items used by the Quechua and other tribes to drink herbal teas. Lapacho is also found in northeast Argentina as the name of a place near Lake Lapacho, about twelve miles west of the city of the Las Palmas in the province of Chaco. See D. A. di Santillan, *Gran Enciclopedia Argentina*, 4 (Buenos Aires: Ediar, 1958), 332.
46. Teodoro Meyer, *Lapachol-Meyer* (San Miguel de Tucuman, Argentina: Foundation Miguel Lillo, undated). Translation.
47. Ibid.
48. Ibid.
49. See note 41 above.
50. See note 34 above.
51. See note 35 above.
52. See note 34 above.
53. Cesar Colombres, San Miguel de Tucuman, Argentina; personal communication, November 1983.
54. See note 34 above.
55. See note 53 above.
56. Oscar Ramon Ahumada, letter to the editor, *La Gazeta* (San Miguel de Tucuman, Argentina), May 10, 1969. Translation.
57. See note 34 above.
58. See note 53 above.

59. "Pau d'Arco (*Tabebuia avellanedae*): Directions to Use," Dr. Adalgiso Volpini, Farmacia N.S. De Siao, São Paulo, Brazil, undated. 1 pg.

CHAPTER TWO

1.   J. Harshberger, "Purposes of Ethnobotany," *Botanical Gazette* 21 (1896): 146–54.
2.   R. E. Schultes, "The Place of Ethnobotany in the Ethnopharmacologic Search for Psychomimetic Drugs" in *Ethnopharmacologic Search for Psychoactive Drugs*, ed., D. Efron (Washington, D.C.: U.S. Government Printing Office, 1967).
3.   Alec de Montmorency, "Ancient South American Cancer Cure Blacked Out in America," *The Spotlight* (Washington, D.C.), January 5, 1981, 11; and "South American Medicine Men Still Cure With Herbal Remedies," *The Spotlight*, March 1981.
4.   Ibid.
5.   A. H. Gentry, "The Cultivated Species of *Tabebuia*," *Florida Nurseryman*, May 1984, 8–10, 39.
6.   Louise Tenney, "Pau d'Arco (*Tabebuia altissima*): What Is New Is Not Necessarily True, What Is True Is Not Necessarily New," *Cancer News Journal* 17 (1982): 26–27.
7.   Louise Tenney, "Taheebo 'An Herb for All Reasons,'" undated, 1 pg.
8.   Louise Tenney, "Pau d'Arco," *Today's Herbs* 3, no. 9 (May 1983): 1–3.
9.   Jerome Godin, "Lapacho and Aveloz: Can They Really Cure Cancer and Other Chronic Conditions?" *Total Health Happenings* 1, no. 3 (May, 1983): 1–3.
10. Brian Power and Nicole Parton, "Cancer 'Cure' Sales Banned," *The Sun* (Vancouver, B.C.), February 14, 1985, A1 and A2.
11. Peter O'Neil, "Tea Bags VSE Action," *The Province* (Vancouver, B.C.), April 24, 1985, 22.
12. W. Martin, "Soy and Breast Cancer," *Townsend Letter for Doctors*, no. 117 (April 1993): 328–29. In 1994, Canadian physicians were highly impressed when pau d' arco combined with radiation in a self-treatment of prostate cancer seemed to cause "early recovery." See Lisa M. Cherry, "To Be Taken Only in an Emergency," *The Globe and Mail* (Toronto), April 22, 1994, A-13.
13. "Pau d'Arco (*Tabebuia avellanedae*): Directions to Use." Dr. Adalgiso Volpini, Farmacia N.S. De Siao, São Paulo, Brazil, undated, 1 pg.
14. R. Anton et al., "Pharmacognosy of *Mimosa tenuiflora* (Willd.) Poiret," *Journal of Ethnopharmacology* 38 (1993): 153–57.
15. M. E. Marti, "Phyto-Active Cosmetics," *Drug and Cosmetic Industry* 150 (1992): 36–46.
16. Editorial, "The Natural Way Ahead?" *Manufacturing Chemist* 60, no. 9 (1989): 33, 40. See also note 15 above.
17. See note 14 above.
18. X. Lozoya et al., "Experimental Evaluation of *Mimosa tenuiflora* (Willd.) Poir. (Tepeschuite). I. Screening of the Antimicrobial Properties of Bark Extracts," *Archivos de Investigacions Medica* (Mexico) 20 (1989): 87–93.
19. E. Carlson, "Synergistic Effect of *Candida albicans* and *Staphylococcus aureus* on Mouse Mortality," *Infection and Immunity* 38 (1982): 921–24.
20. C. Anesini and C. Perez, "Screening of Plants Used in Argentine Folk Medicine

for Antimicrobial Activity," *Journal of Ethnopharmacology* 39 (1993): 119–28.

21. W. C. Wilson, *The Tannic Acid Treatment of Burns*, Great Britain Medical Research Council, Special Report Series, no. 141 (London: His Majesty's Stationary Office, 1929), 1–14.

22. *Scientific Literature Reviews on Generally Recognized As Safe (GRAS) Food Ingredients—Tannic Acid.* (Springfield, Virginia: National Technical Information Service, U.S. Department of Commerce, July 1973), 1.

23. Gail Nielsen, *Candida* Research and Information Foundation (CIRF), Castro Valley, California; personal communication, July 1983.

24. Ibid.

25. Daniel Herman, "The Lapacho, a New Treatment for *Candida albicans,*" *The Environmental Illness Association Newsletter*, February/March 1983, 6–7.

26. C. O. Truss, "Tissue Injury by *Candida albicans.* Mental and Neurological Manifestations," *Orthomolecular Psychiatry* 7 (1978): 17–37.

27. Shirley S. Lorenzani, Ph.D., "*Candida albicans*: Is This Strain of Yeast Friend or Foe?" *Let's Live* (April 1983): 16, 18, 22.

28. Robert E. Foreman, Ph.D., "*Candida albicans*: A Lingering Problem," *Let's Live* (February 1984): 49–50.

29. Ibid.

30. See note 26 above.

31. S. E. Straus, "The Chronic Mononucleosis Syndrome," *Infectious Diseases* 157 (1988): 405–12.

32. S. E. Straus et al., "Allergy and the Chronic Fatigue Syndrome," *Journal of Allergy and Chemical Immunology* 81, part 1 (1988): 791–95.

33. C. O. Truss, "The Role of *Candida albicans* in Human Illness," *Orthomolecular Psychiatry* 10 (1981): 228–38.

34. Gail Nielsen; personal communication, April 1992.

35. "Endoplex 5" and "Allerplex 2" in *Herb Technology*, catalog, 11, 15. Herb Technology, 1305 N.E. 45th St., #205, Seattle, WA 98105.

36. William G. Crook, M.D., *Chronic Fatigue Syndrome and the Yeast Connection.* (Jackson, Tennessee: Professional Books, 1992). See also E. J. Conley, "Treatment of HHV-6 Reactivation in CFIDS," *CFIDS Chronicle Physicians' Forum*, Fall 1993, 15–17. The preliminary results of a study by Dr. E. J. Conley found "a large percentage" of his chronic fatigue syndrome patients showing significant elevations in antibody readings for *Candida*, indicating *Candida* overgrowth. This finding may bear upon acute inflammatory reactions to *C. albicans* in women with recurrent vaginal yeast infections. These reactions have recently been associated with the overactivity of an immune system component also known to be activated in inflammatory arthritis. See R. B. Ashman et al., "Association of a Complement Allotype (C3F) with Acute Inflammatory Responses to *Candida albicans* Infection," *Medical Journal of Australia* 160 (1994): 732-33. If further associations are established in patients with yeast syndrome, the syndrome might become classified as an autoimmune disorder.

37. See notes 31 and 32 above.

38. See note 28 above.

39. Martin H. Zwerling et al., "The Expanding Spectrum of Candidiasis," *Health World* magazine (April/May 1992): 10–13.

40. See note 27 above.

41. D. S. Bauman and H. E. Hagglund, "Correlation between Certain Polysystem

Chronic Complaints and an Enzyme Immunoassay with Antigens of *Candida albicans*," *Journal of Advancement in Medicine* 4 (1991): 5–9. Immunoassay from Progena, P.O. Box 14493, Albuquerque, NM 87191.

42. *Candida Research and Information Foundation Newsletter* (July 1984). P.O. Box 2719, Castro Valley, CA 94546.

43. The Environmental Illness Association, P.O. Box 5003, Berkeley, CA 94705.

44. The Human Ecology Foundation, Head Office, 465 Highway 8, Dundas, Ontario L9H 4V9, Canada.

45. C. Orion Truss, M.D., *The Missing Diagnosis*, 1983. The Missing Diagnosis, P.O. Box 26508, Birmingham, AL 35226.

46. William G. Crook, M.D. *The Yeast Connection,* (Jackson, Tenn.: Professional Books, 1983).

47. Andrew Nikiforuk and Barbara Binczyk, "The Pariah Syndrome," *Harrowsmith* (August/September, 1982): 51–60.

48. Richard Leviton, "Environmental Illness: A Special Report," *Yoga Journal* (November/December, 1990): 43–53, 95–100.

49. Gary R. Oberg, M.D., *An Overview of the Philosophy of the American Academy of Environmental Medicine* (Denver, Colorado: American Academy of Environmental Medicine, 1992), 5–6. See also Theron G. Randolph, M.D., *Environmental Medicine—Beginnings and Bibliographies of Clinical Ecology* (Fort Collins, Colorado: Clinical Ecology Publications, 1987), and William J. Rea, M.D., *Chemical Sensitivity—Volume 1* (Chelsea, Michigan: Lewis Publishers, 1993); and N. Senanayake and G. C. Roman, "Disorders of Neuromuscular Transmission Due to Natural Environmental Toxins," *Journal of the Neurological Sciences* 107 (1992): 1-13.

50. Stephen H. Hall, "Allergic to the 20th Century," *Health* (May/June 1993): 72–80, 85. See also V. Carpman, "Chemical Warfare: CFIDS, Multiple Chemical Sensitivity and Silicone Implant Disorder, " *CFIDS Chronicle Physicians' Forum* (Fall 1993): 33-34.

51. See note 48 above.

52. See note 50 above.

53. See note 48 above.

54. L. Renfro et al., "Yeast Connection among 100 Patients with Chronic Fatigue," *American Journal of Medicine* 86 (1989): 165–68.

55. See notes 48 and 49 above.

56. See note 42 above.

57. See notes 47–49 above.

58. Lois Ember, "Study Confirms Paucity of Chemical Toxicity Data," *Chemical and Engineering News* (March 12, 1984): 12.

59. Earon S. Davis, J.D., M.P.H., letter to the editor, *Townsend Letter for Doctors*, no. 95 (June 1991): 447–48.

60. American College of Physicians, "Position Paper on Clinical Ecology," *Annals of Internal Medicine* 111 (1989): 168–78.

61. Donald W. Black, M.D., University of Iowa College of Medicine, letter to the editor, *Townsend Letter for Doctors* , no. 95 (June 1991): 447–48.

62. See note 59 above.

63. Rona Maynard, "The Allergy Nightmare of Sandra Stronge," *Chatelaine* (April 1985): 68, 84, 86, 88–89, 95–96. See also notes 47 and 50 above.

64. Michael A. Weiner, *Maximum Immunity* (Boston: Houghton Mifflin, 1986), 241.

65. Gail Nielsen; personal communication, November 1984.
66. See note 46 above.
67. See note 64 above.
68. See note 42 above.
69. See note 65 above.
70. See notes 23 and 25 aboe.
71. See note 23 above.
72. See note 65 above.
73. Gail Nielsen, "LaPacho: An Herbal Alternative?" *The Human Ecologist*, no. 22 (Summer 1983): 12–13.
74. *Candida Research and Information Foundation Newsletter*, no. 9/10 (March 1989): 8–10.
75. See note 65 above.
76. See note 25 above.
77. See note 73 above.
78. See note 33 above.
79. See note 74 above.
80. See note 25 above.
81. See note 23 above.
82. See note 42 above.
83. J. G. Alexander, "Allergy in the Gastrointestinal Tract," *The Lancet* 2 (December 20, 1975): 1264.
84. J. W. Rippon, *Medical Mycology*, third edition (Philadelphia: W. B. Saunders, 1988), 557.
85. *Candida Research and Information Foundation Newsletter* (October 1984): 16.
86. M. W. DeGregorio et al., "*Candida* Infections in Patients with Acute Leukemia: Ineffectiveness of Nystatin Prophylaxis and Relationship between Oropharyngeal and Systemic Candidiasis," *Cancer* 50 (1982): 2780–84.
87. D. Armstrong, "Fungemia in the Immunocompromised Host: Changing Patterns, Antigenemia, High Mortality," *American Journal of Medicine* 71 (1981): 363–70.
88. J. S. Solomkin et al., "*Candida* Infections in Surgical Patients: Dose Requirements and Toxicity of Amphotericin B," *Annals of Surgery* 195 (1982): 177–85.
89. John Parks Trowbridge, M.D., and Morton Walker, D.P.M., *The Yeast Syndrome* (New York: Bantam Books, 1986), 339.
90. A. S. Rosenberg and A. E. Brown, "Infection in the Cancer Patient," *Disease-a-Month* 39 (1993): 511–17, 529.
91. Ibid.
92. J. D. Stobo et al., "Suppressor Thymus-Derived Lymphocytes in Fungal Infection," *Journal of Clinical Investigation* 57 (1976): 319–28.
93. See note 31 above.
94. Trowbridge and Walker, *Yeast Syndrome*, 292–93.
95. See note 32 above.
96. S. S. Witkin et al., "Inhibition of *Candida albicans*–Induced Lymphocyte Proliferation by Lymphocytes and Sera from Women with Recurrent Vaginitis," *American Journal of Obstetrics and Gynecology* 147 (1983): 809–11.
97. R. D. Nelson et al., "Two Mechanisms of Inhibition of Human Lymphocyte Proliferation by Soluble Yeast Mannan Polysaccharide," *Infection and Immunity* 43 (1984): 1041–46.

98. L. Romani et al., "Neutralizing Antibody to Interleukin 4 Induces Systemic Protection and T Helper Type 1–Associated Immunity in Murine Candidiasis," *Journal of Experimental Medicine* 176 (1992): 19–25.

99. T. G. Sieck et al., "Protection against Murine Disseminated Candidiasis Mediated by a *Candida albicans*–Specific T-Cell Line," *Infection and Immunity* 61 (1993): 3540–43.

100. News release, National Institutes of Health, "Immune Abnormalities Found in Chronic Fatigue Syndrome May Lead to Better Understanding of the Disease," *Townsend Letter for Doctors*, no. 118 (May, 1993): 504.

101. S. E. Straus et al., "Lymphocyte Phenotype and Function in the Chronic Fatigue Syndrome," *Journal of Clinical Immunology* 73 (1993): 30–40.

102. See notes 100 and 101 above.

103. See note 3 above.

104. Jônio de Freitas Mota and Manoel Motta, "A Conspiraçao do Silêncio," *O'Cruzeiro* (São Paulo), March 25, 1967. Translation.

105. *Candida Research and Information Foundation Newsletter*, no. 11/12 (July 1990): 7.

106. Octaviano Gaiarsa, "Estudos e Microscopia do Ipé Roxo Ede Outras Especies Vegetais." Santo André, São Paulo, Brazil, 1968, unpublished, 12 pages. Translation.

107. Janis B. Alcorn, *Huastec Mayan Ethnobotany* (Austin: University of Texas Press, 1984), 802.

108. Octaviano Gaiarsa, Santo André, São Paulo; letter to the author, October 2, 1983.

109. W. Donald MacRae, Ph.D., then at the Department of Botany, University of British Columbia, Vancouver, B.C.; personal communication, September 1983.

110. Barbara Dickey, Critical Illness Research Foundation Laboratory, Birmingham, Alabama; personal communication, February 1984.

111. Ibid.

112. H. Wagner et al., "Immunological Investigations of Naphthoquinone-Containing Plant Extracts, Isolated Quinones and other Cytostatic Compounds in Cellular Immunosystems," *Planta Medica*, no. 6 (1986): 550-A. Poster.

113. B. Kreher et al., "New Furanonaphthoquinones and other Constituents of *Tabebuia avellanedae* and Their Immunomodulating Activities *in Vitro*," *Planta Medica* 54, no. 6 (1988): 562. Poster.

114. J. Wesley Alexander and Robert A. Good, eds., *Clinical Immunology* (Philadelphia: W.B. Saunders Company, 1977), 196–97.

115. A. Polak and P. G. Hartman, "Antifungal Chemotherapy—Are We Winning?" *Progress in Drug Research*, 37. (1991): 227–29.

116. Daniel P. Mowrey, Lehi, Utah; personal communication, May 1992.

117. Mark Konlee, "Keep Hope Alive," Franklin, Wisconsin; letter to the editor, *Townsend Letter for Doctors*, no. 95 (June 1991): 444–46.

CHAPTER THREE

1. Samuel J. Record and Clayton D. Mell, *Timbers of Tropical America* (New Haven, Conn.: Yale University Press, 1924), 538–42.

2. S. J. Record and R. W. Hess, "American Timbers of the Family Bignoniaceae," *Tropical Woods*, no. 63 (1940): 9–38. Record and Hess gave the main species of the pau d'arco group as *Tabebuia serratifolia*, *T. heptaphylla* (=*T. ipe*),

T. impetiginosa (=*T. palmeri*), and *T. barbata*. For the purpose of brevity, I have used the name "pau d'arco" more broadly to include any *Tabebuia* used in folk medicine.

3. Samuel J. Record and Robert W. Hess, *Timbers of the New World* (New Haven, Conn.: Yale University Press, 1943), 86.

4. Jônio de Freitas Mota and Manoel Motta, "Casos Positivos Comprovam: Descoberta a Cura do Câncer," *O'Cruzeiro* (São Paulo), March 18, 1967. Translation.

5. James A. Taylor, *A Portuguese-English Dictionary*, revised (Stanford, Calif.: Stanford University Press, 1970).

6. Valter Accorsi, University of São Paulo; letter to the author, May 27, 1983.

7. Record and Mell, *Timbers*, 540.

8. See note 5 above. The name pau d'arco is found as a prefix in other plant names designating trees used to make bows. However, by itself the name is commonly applied to *Tabebuia impetiginosa*. See Grande *Enciclopédia Portuguesa e Brasileira* 20 (Lisbon and Rio de Janeiro: Editorial Enciclopédia, 1936–1960), 654.

9. Dennis Werner, *Amazon Journey* (New York: Simon and Schuster, 1984), 21.

10. J. H. Steward, ed., *Handbook of South American Indians I* (Washington, D.C.: U.S. Government Printing Office, 1948): 513-15.

11. A. H. Gentry, "Bignoniaceae—Part I," *Flora Neotropica*, monograph 25 (1980): 44-47.

12. M. Chudnoff, *Tropical Timbers of the World* (Madison, Wis.: United States Department of Agriculture, Forest Service, Forest Products Laboratory, April 1980), 293–94.

13. Alwyn H. Gentry was featured in an article by Peter T. White in *National Geographic*, January 1983, titled "Tropical Rain Forests: Nature's Dwindling Treasures," 2–47.

14. See note 11 above.

15. See note 12 above.

16. See note 2 above.

17. See note 1 above.

18. Record and Mell, *Timbers*, 537–39.

19. Teodoro Meyer, "Progresso de los Estudios en el Campo de la Flora del Norests Argentino, desde 1937 hasta la Fecha," *Conference of the Ministry of Education and Justice* (Tucuman, Argentina: Foundation Miguel Lillo, October 23, 1966). Translation.

20. See note 11 above.

21. Thomas H. Everett, *Living Trees of the World* (New York: Chanticleer Press/ Doubleday and Company, 1968), 297–302.

22. Alwyn H. Gentry, "A Synopsis of Bignoniaceae Ethnobotany and Economic Botany," *Annals of the Missouri Botanical Garden* 79 (1992): 53–64.

23. M. Lozoya-Meckes and V. Mellado-Campos, "Is the *Tecoma stans* Infusion an Antidiabetic Remedy?" *Journal of Ethnopharmacology* 14 (1985): 1–9.

24. Kenneth Jones, "Tronadora: Antidiabetic Plant of Mexico," *Townsend Letter for Doctors*, no. 124 (November 1993): 1066–67.

25. G. G. Colin, "Study on the Anti-Diabetic Properties of *Tecoma mollis*. Preliminary Report," *Journal of the American Pharmaceutical Association* 15 (1926): 556–60.

26. Julia F. Morton, *Atlas of Medicinal Plants of Middle America* (Springfield, Ill.:

Charles C Thomas Publishers, 1981), 829–32.

27. F. O. Bobbio et al., "Identification of a Peonidin-3-cinnamylsophoroside in the Flowers of *Tabebuia impetiginosa*," *HortScience* 23 (1988): 1089.

28. E.A. Menninger, "*Tabebuia* Trees for Warm Regions," *Journal of the New York Botanical Garden* 50 (1949): 121–29.

29. Alwyn H. Gentry, "The Cultivated Species of *Tabebuia*," *Florida Nurseryman* 31 (1984): 8–10, 39.

30. See note 2 above.

31. See note 6 above.

32. N. J. Turner and R. J. Hebda, "Contemporary Use of Bark for Medicine by Two Salishan Native Elders of Southeast Vancouver Island, Canada," *Journal of Ethnopharmacology* 29 (1990): 59–72.

33. Teodoro Meyer, San Miguel de Tucuman, Argentina; letter to the author, February 12, 1984.

34. See note 6 above.

35. Alwyn H. Gentry, Missouri Botanical Garden; personal communication, March 1984.

36. See note 22 above.

37. See note 35 above.

38. I. S. Wright and L. M. Nekhom, *Historical Dictionary of Argentina* (Metuchen, N.J., and London: The Scarecrow Press, 1978): 66.

39. Alwyn H. Gentry, *Bignoniaceae—Part II (Tribe Tecomeae). Flora Neotropica*, monograph 25, part 2 (New York: New York Botanical Garden, 1992), 249–51.

40. See note 35 above.

41. Morton, *Atlas*, 828–29.

42. James A. Duke and K. Wain, "Medicinal Plants of the World" (Beltsville, Md.: unpublished computerized index).

43. J. Jui, "A Survey of Some Medicinal Plants of Mexico for Selected Biological Activities," *Journal of Natural Products* 29 (1966): 250–259.

44. See note 42 above.

45. Hernando Garcia Barriga, *Flora Medicinal De Colombia. Botanica Medica* (Bogota, Colombia: Instituto de Ciencias Naturales, Universidad Nacional, 1975), 145–50. Translation.

46. See note 43 above.

47. "Tannic Acid" entry in *Martindale's: The Extra Pharmacopoeia*, 28th ed. James E. F. Reynolds, ed. (London: Pharmaceutical Press, 1982), 287.

48. R. Wasicky, et al., "Fitoquímica de *Tabebuia* sp. ("Ipê Roxo"): 1—Analise de Alguns Princípios," *Revista da Faculade de Farmácia e Bioquimica da Universidade de São Paulo* 5 (1967): 383–95. Translation.

49. Joachim Kühnau, "The Flavonoids. A Class of Semi-Essential Food Components: Their Role in Human Nutrition." *World Review of Nutrition and Dietetics*, 24 (1976): 117–91.

50. *Merck Index*, 9th ed. (Rahway, N.J.: Merck and Company, 1976), 243.

51. G. I. Forrest and D. S. Bendall, "The Distribution of Polyphenols in the Tea Plant (*Camellia sinensis* L.)," *Biochemical Journal* 113 (1969): 741–55.

52. R. S. Thompson et al., "Plant Proanthocyanidins. Part I. Introduction; The Isolation, Structure, and Distribution in Nature of Plant Procyanidins," *Journal of the Chemical Society, Perkin Transactions* 1 (1972): 1387–99.

53. See note 49 above.

54. E. Alonso, et al., "Suitability of Water/Ethanol Mixtures for the Extraction of Catechins and Proanthocyanidins from *Vitis vinifera* Seeds Contained in a Winery By-Product," *Seed Science and Technology* 19 (1991): 545–52.
55. G. Proserpio, "Natural Sunscreens: Vegetable Derivatives As Sunscreens and Tanning Agents," *Cosmetics and Toiletries* 91 (March 1976): 34–46.
56. E. Stahl and I. Ittel," Natürliche UV-Filter für Sonnenschultzmittel," *Parfümerie und Kosmetik* 62, no. 4 (1981): 8 pp. Translation.
57. See note 49 above.
58. Ibid.
59. T. J. Haley et al., "Studies on 'Vitamin P.' I. Topically Applied Vitamin P-like Substances on the Mammalian Capillary Bed," *Proceedings of the Society for Experimental Biology and Medicine* 64 (1947): 202–7.
60. T. Okuda et al., "Studies on the Activities of Tannins and Related Compounds from Medicinal Plants and Drugs. I. Inhibitory Effects on Lipid Peroxidation in Mitochondria and Microsomes of Liver," *Chemical and Pharmaceutical Bulletin* 31 (1983): 1625–31.
61. A. Salama and C. Mueller-Eckhardt, "Cianidanol and Its Metabolites Bind Tightly to Red Blood Cells and Are Responsible for the Production of Auto- and/or Drug-Dependant Antibodies Against These Cells," *British Journal of Haematology* 66 (1987): 263–66.
62. See note 59 above.
63. M. M. de Oliveira et al., "Antitumor Activity of Condensed Flavanols," *Anais Academia Brasileira de Ciencias* 44 (1972): 41–44.
64. H. H. S. Fong et al., "Antitumor Activity of Certain Plants Due to Tannins," *Journal of Pharmaceutical Sciences* 61 (1972): 1818.
65. N. Kakiuchi et al., "Inhibiting Effect of Tannins on Reverse Transcriptase from RNA Tumor Virus," *Journal of Natural Products* 48 (1985): 614–21.
66. Jane E. Brody, "Scientists Seeking Possible Wonder Drugs in Tea," *The New York Times*, March 14, 1991.
67. T. Kada et al., "Detection and Chemical Identification of Natural Bio-antimutagens: A Case of the Green Tea Factor," *Mutation Research* 150 (1985): 127–32. See also H. Mukhtar et al., "Tea Components: Antimutagenic and Anticarcinogenic Effects," *Preventive Medicine* 21 (1992): 351–60.
68. K. Muramatsu et al., "Effect of Green Tea Catechins on Plasma Cholesterol Level in Cholesterol-Fed Rats," *Journal of Nutrition and Science Vitaminology* 32 (1986): 613–22.
69. N. Horiba et al., "A Pilot Study of Japanese Green Tea As a Medicament: Antibacterial and Bactericidal Effects," *Journal of Endodontics* 17 (1991): 122–24.
70. I. Morel et al., "Antioxidant and Iron-chelating Activities of the Flavonoids Catechin, Quercetin and Diosmetin on Iron-loaded Rat Hepatocyte Cultures," *Biochemical Pharmacology* 45 (1993): 13–19.
71. H. P. T. Ammon and M. Handel, "Crataegus Toxicologie und Pharmacologie Teil II: Pharmakodynamik," *Planta Medica* 43 (1981): 209–39.
72. B. Zhao et al., "Scavenging Effect of Extracts of Green Tea and Natural Antioxidants on Active Oxygen Radicals," *Cell Biophysics* 14 (1989): 175 (abstract).
73. Y. Sagesaka-Mitane et al., "Platelet Aggregation Inhibitors in Hot Water Extract of Green Tea," *Chemical and Pharmaceutical Bulletin* 38 (1990): 790–93. See also M. G. L. Hertog et al.,"Dietary Antioxidant Flavonoids and Risk

of Coronary Heart Disease: The Zutphen Elderly Study," *The Lancet 342* (October 23, 1993): 1007-11.

74. Z. Y. Wang et al., "Interaction of Epicatechins Derived from Green Tea with Rat Hepatic Cytochrome P-450," *Drug Metabolism and Disposition* 16 (1988): 98.
75. See note 63 above.
76. Gentry, *Bignoniaceae—Part II*, 144–45.
77. See note 63 above.
78. N. M. Ferguson and E. J. Lien, "A Flavonol Rutinoside from *Tecoma ipe* Flava (Pau d'Arco)," *Oriental Healing Arts International Bulletin* 13 (1988): 184–86.
79. N. M. Ferguson and E. J. Lien, "An Isolated Glucoside from *Tecoma ipe* Rosa," *Oriental Healing Arts Bulletin* 13 (1988): 187–88.
80. See note 27 above.
81. A. B. Pomilio and J. F. Sproviero, "Anthocyanins from Argentine *Tabebuia* Species," *Phytochemistry* 10 (1971): 1399–1400.
82. K. Odake et al., "Chemical Structures of Two Anthocyanins from Purple Sweet Potato, *Ipomoea batatas*," *Phytochemistry* 31 (1992): 2127–30.
83. See note 48 above.
84. J. M. Riddle, "Ancient and Medieval Chemotherapy for Cancer," *ISIS* 76 (1985): 319–30.
85. Janis B. Alcorn, New Orleans, Louisiana; personal communication, July 1985.
86. Janis B. Alcorn; letter to the author, July 11, 1985.
87. Ibid.
88. Janis B. Alcorn, *Huastec Mayan Ethnobotany*, (Austin: University of Texas Press, 1984), 802.
89. X. A. Dominguez and J. B. Alcorn, "Screening of Medicinal Plants Used by Huastec Mayans of Northeastern Mexico," *Journal of Ethnopharmacology* 13 (1985): 139–56.
90. See note 88 above.
91. See note 86 above.
92. E. Messer, "The Hot and Cold in Mesoamerican Indigenous and Hispanicized Thought," *Social Science and Medicine* 25 (1987): 339-46.
93. See notes 86 and 89 above.
94. See note 89 above.
95. See note 86 above.
96. See note 89 above.
97. See note 84 above.
98. See note 89 above.
99. See note 86 above.
100. J. C. Th. Uphof, *Dictionary of Economic Plants*, 2nd ed. (New York: Verlag von J. Cramer, 1968), 115.
101. Morton, *Atlas*, 142–43.
102. Richard A. Rutter, *Catalogo De Plantas Utiles De La Amazonia Peruana* (Yarinacocha, Pucallpa, Peru: Ministerio de Educacion, Instituto Lingüistica de Verano, 1990), 51–52.
103. See notes 86, 88, and 89 above.
104. Rutter, *Catalogo*, 54–55.
105. R. E. Schultes, "De Plantas Toxicariis E Mundo Novo Tropicale Commentationes XXVI: Ethnopharmacological Notes on the Flora of Northwestern South

America," *Botanical Museum Leaflets Harvard University* 28 (1980): 34.
106. Morton, *Atlas*, 789–90.
107. Rutter, *Catalogo*, 173.
108. Morton, *Atlas*, 825.
109. See notes 86 and 89 above.
110. Uphof, *Dictionary*, 412, 116.
111. Morton, *Atlas*, 340–41.
112. See note 110 above.
113. Rutter, *Catalogo*, 52.
114. See note 88 above.
115. Morton, *Atlas*, 401–3.
116. Uphof, *Dictionary*, 524.
117. I. M. Grundy and B. M. Campbell, "Potential Production and Utilization of Oil from *Trichilia* spp. (Meliaceae)," *Economic Botany* 47 (1993): 148–53.
118. Morton, *Atlas*, 407–8.
119. See note 89 above.
120. Rutter, *Catalogo*, 78.
121. Walter H. Lewis and Memory P. F. Elvin-Lewis, *Medical Botany* (New York: John Wiley, 1977), 259.
122. Nicole Maxwell, *Witch Doctor's Apprentice*, 3rd ed. (New York: Citadel Press, 1990), 293, 390.
123. P. R. Bergstresser et al., "Dendritic Epidermal T-Cells: Lessons from Mice for Humans," *Journal of Investigative Dermatology* 100, suppl. 1 (1993): 805–35.
124. K. Danno, "Immunomodulatory Effect by Ultraviolet Light: Dual Regulation of Cutaneous Immune Cell Functions," *Acta Dermatologia* (Kyoto) 87 (1993): 575–85.
125. R. L. Edelson and J. M. Fink, "The Immunological Function of Skin," *Scientific American* 252 (June 1985): 46–53.
126. T. Izumoto et al., "Relationship between Transference of a Drug from a Transdermal Patch and the Physiochemical Properties," *Chemical and Pharmaceutical Bulletin* 40 (1992): 456–58.
127. M. Iguchi et al., "Homeostasis As Regulated by Activated Macrophage. V. Suppression of Diabetes Mellitus in Non-obese Diabetic Mice by LPSw from Wheat Flour," *Chemical and Pharmaceutical Bulletin* 40 (1992): 1004–6. See also "The Pores Have It," *HerbalGram* no. 22 (Spring 1990): 41; and C. Portera, "Skin-Deep Water Worries," *Longevity* (August 1994): 26.
128. Gentry, *Bignoniaceae—Part II*, 145–46.
129. Morton, *Atlas*, 827–28.
130. See note 128 above.
131. See note 129 above.
132. S. A. McClure and W. H. Eshbaugh, "Love Potions of Andros Island, Bahamas," *Journal of Ethnobiology* 3 (1983): 149–56.
133. E. Elizabetsky et al., "Traditional Amazonian Nerve Tonics As Antidepressant Agents: *Chaunochiton kappleri*: A Case Study," *Journal of Herbs, Spices and Medicinal Plants* 1 (1992): 125-62.
134. See note 128 above.
135. See note 129 above.
136. Morton, *Atlas*, 707–8.
137. Siri von Reis Altschul, *Drugs and Foods from Little-Known Plants: Notes in

Harvard University Herbaria (Cambridge, Mass.: Harvard University Press, 1973), 274.

138. Gentry, Bignoniaceae—Part II, pp. 254–58.
139. See note 11 above.
140. Alwyn H. Gentry; personal communication, February 1984.
141. Ibid.
142. Valter Accorsi, University of São Paulo; personal communication, May 1983.
143. Fadlo Fraige Filho, São Paulo; personal communication, June 1983.
144. M. A. G. e Barros, "Flora Medicinal Do Distrito Federal," Brasil Florestal 12 (1982): 35–45. The "Ipé-amarelo" given is Tabebuia caraiba (Mart.) Bur., for which Gentry, in Bignoniaceae—Part II, p. 144, gives the correct species as T. aurea (Manso) Bentham and Hooker f. ex S. Moore.
145. B. M. Boom and S. Moestl, "Ethnobotanical Notes of José M. Cruxant from the Franco-Venezuelan Expedition to the Headwaters of the Orinoco River, 1951–1952," Economic Botany 44 (1990): 416–19.
146. Gentry, Bignoniaceae—Part II, 204–7.
147. W. Wilbert and G. Haiek, "Phytochemical Screening of a Warao Pharmacopoeia Employed to Treat Gastrointestinal Disorders," Journal of Ethnopharmacology 34 (1991): 7–11. See also note 35 above, in which Gentry states that the closely related Tabebuia insignis var. monophylla sandw. has been used "to treat conjunctivitis."
148. Richard Evans Schultes and Robert F. Raffauf, The Healing Forest: Medicinal and Toxic Plants of the Northwest Amazonia (Portland, Ore.: Dioscorides Press, 1990), 107–8.
149. Gentry, Bignoniaceae—Part II, 206–7.
150. James A. Duke, "Tabebuia spp. (Bignoniaceae) Pao d'arco," unpublished, 1983, 4 pp. See also James A Duke and Rodolfo Vasquez, Amazonian Ethnobotanical Dictionary (Boca Raton, Fl.: CRC Press, 1994): 164.
151. See note 45 above.
152. E. W. Davis, "The Ethnobotany of Chamairo: Mussatia hyacintha," Journal of Ethnopharmacology 9 (1983): 225–36.
153. Isabel Vincent, "Getting 'Well' Where Incas Once Dwelled," The Globe and Mail (Toronto), March 21, 1992, A9.
154. J. W. Bastien, "Herbal Curing by Quollahuaya Andeans," Journal of Ethnopharmacology 8 (1983): 13–28.
155. See note 153 above.
156. See note 154 above.
157. J. W. Bastien, "Pharmacopeia of Qollahuaya Andeans," Journal of Ethnopharmacology 8 (1983): 97–111.
158. Joseph W. Bastien, University of Texas at Arlington; personal communication, March 1984.
159. See note 157 above.
160. Joseph W. Bastien, Healers of the Andes: Kallawaya Herbalists and Their Medicinal Plants (Salt Lake City: University of Utah Press, 1987), 14–17.
161. Ibid.
162. Ibid., 22–24.
163. Ibid.
164. See note 160 above.
165. See note 162 above.
166. See notes 160 and 162 above.

167. Ibid., 38–55.
168. Joseph W. Bastien, *Drum and Stethoscope: Integrating Ethnomedicine and Biomedicine in Bolivia* (Salt Lake City: University of Utah Press, 1992), 47.
169. See note 157 above.
170. Ibid., 229.
171. Bastien, *Healers of the Andes*, 64.
172. See notes 154 and 158 above.
173. See note 157 above.
174. Gentry, *Bignoniaceae—Part II*, 257, 247, 227, 192.
175. See note 158 above.
176. See note 154 above.
177. Bastien, *Healers of the Andes*, 65–66.
178. See note 171 above.
179. Ibid.,156.
180. Ibid.
181. "Nettle Cure," *American Herb Association Quarterly Newsletter* 4 (1988): 15.
182. F. Willer and H. Wagner, "Immunologically Active Polysaccharides and Lectins from the Aqueous Extract of *Urtica dioica*," *Planta Medica* 56 (1990): 669. Poster.
183. P. Mittman, "Randomized, Double-Blind Study of Freeze-Dried *Urtica dioica* in the Treatment of Allergic Rhinitis," *Planta Medica* 56 (1990): 44–47.
184. J. Balazarin et al., "The Mannose-Specific Plant Lectins from *Cymbidium* Hybrid and *Epiactis helleborine* and the (*N*-acetylglucosamide) N-Specific Plant Lectin from *Urtica dioica* Are Potent Selective Inhibitors of Human Immunodeficiency Virus and Cytomegalovirus Replication in Vitro," *Antiviral Research* 18 (1992): 191–207.
185. I. B. Quieroz and S. L. Reis, "Antispasmodic and Analgesic Effects of Some Medicinal Plants," *Brazilian-Sino Symposium on Chemistry and Pharmacology of Natural Products*, Rio de Janeiro, December 10–14, 1989 (Ministry of State, Foundation Oswaldo Cruz), poster 180, p. 246.
186. M. Markov, "On the Pharmacology of *Plantago major*," *Second International Congress on Ethnopharmacology*, Uppsala, Sweden, July 2–4, 1992 (Swedish Academy of Pharmaceutical Sciences), poster 6.
187. M. Matev et al., "Clinical Trial of *Plantago major* Preparation in the Treatment of Chronic Bronchitis," *Vutreshni Bolesti (Sofia)* 21 (1982): 133–37 (in Russian).
188. See note 171 above.
189. P. A. G. M. de Smet, "An Introduction to Herbal Pharmacoepidemiology," *Journal of Ethnopharmacology* 38 (1993): 197–208.
190. A. Scarpa and A. Aimi, "The Ethnomedical Study of *Soroche* (i.e., Altitude Sickness) in the Andean Plateaus of Peru," *Fitoterapia* 52 (1981): 147–64. Scarpa and Aimi list *Tecoma grandiceps*, which Gentry, in the following reference, identifies correctly as *Tabebuia ochracea* ssp. *ochracea*.
191. Gentry, *Bignoniaceae—Part II*, 226–30.
192. C. S. Houston, "Mountain Sickness," *Scientific American* (October 1992): 58–66.
193. See note 190 above.
194. Rutter, *Catalogo*, 238; Rutter gives *Tecoma caraiba* and *Tecoma conspicua*, species that Gentry identifies correctly as *Tabebuia aurea* (see note 76 above) and *Tabebuia serratifolia* (see note 138 above).

195. C. F. Spencer et al., "Survey of Plants for Antimalarial Activity," *Lloydia* 10 (1947): 145–74. See also note 144 above.

196. Ibid.

197. See notes 138, 192, and 194 above.

198. Carlos Reynel et al., *Etnobotanica Campa-Ashaninca* (Lima, Peru: Universidad Nacional Agraria La Mollina, 1990), 55, 75–76. Translation.

199. J. L. Hartwell, "Plants Used Against Cancer: A Survey," *Lloydia* 32 (1968): 153–205.

200. S. M. Kupchan et al., "Tumor Inhibitors. VIII. Eupatorin, New Cytotoxic Flavone from *Eupatorium semiserratum*," *Journal of Pharmaceutical Sciences* 54 (1965): 929–30.

201. O. Sticher, "Plant Mono-, Di and Sesquiterpenoids with Pharmacological or Therapeutical Activity" in *New Natural Products and Plant Drugs with Pharmacological, Biological, or Therapeutical Activity*, eds., H. Wagner and P. Wolff. (Berlin: Springer-Verlag, 1977), 137–76.

202. N. T. D. Trang et al., "Thymoquinone from *Eupatorium ayapana*," *Planta Medica* 59 (1993): 99.

203. D. Bamba et al., "Essential Oil of *Eupatorium odoratum*," *Planta Medica* 59 (1993): 184–85.

204. Morton, *Atlas*, 931.

205. I. H. Hall et al., "Anti-Inflammatory Activity of Sesquiterpene Lactones and Related Compounds," *Journal of Pharmaceutical Sciences* 68 (1979): 537–42.

206. C. C. Culvenor, "Tumor-Inhibitory Activity of Pyrrolizidine Alkaloids," *Journal of Pharmaceutical Sciences* 57 (1968): 1112–17.

207. W. Y. Li and E. J. Lien, "A Survey of Chinese Anticancer Herbs: 1 *Crotalaria sessiflora* L. (*Nung-Chi-Li*) and Pyrrolizidine Alkaloids," *Bulletin of the Oriental Healing Arts Institute of U.S.A.* 9 (1984): 321–32.

208. G. R. Pettit et al., "Antineoplastic Agents, 177. Isolation and Structure of Phyllanthostatin 6," *Journal of Natural Products* 53 (1990): 1406–13.

209. Gordon Cragg, Ph.D., Frederick Cancer Research and Development Center, Frederick, Maryland; personal communication, February 1993.

210. G. R. Pettit et al., "Antineoplastic Agents. 104. Isolation and Structure of the *Phyllanthus acuminatus* Vahl. (Euphorbiaceae) Glycosides," *Journal of Organic Chemistry* 49 (1984): 4258–66.

211. See note 208 above.

212. Uphof, *Dictionary*, 403.

213. D. W. Unander et al., "Uses and Bioassays in *Phyllanthus* (Euphorbiaceae): A Compilation. II. The Subgenus *Phyllanthus*," *Journal of Ethnopharmacology* 34 (1991): 97–133.

214. See note 144 above.

215. J. Eldridge, "Bush Medicine in the Exumas and Long Island, Bahamas: A Field Study," *Economic Botany* 29 (1975): 307–32.

216. See note 213 above.

217. David W. Unander, Department of Biology, Eastern College, St. Davids, Pennsylvania; personal communication, August 6, 1993.

218. K. V. Syamasundra et al., "Antihepatotoxic Principles of *Phyllanthus niruri* Herbs," *Journal of Ethnopharmacology* 14 (1985): 41–44. In India, budhatri (*P. niruri*) is traditionally used to cure coughing, extreme thirst, anemia, and tuberculosis; see V. B. Dash and K. K. Gupta, *Materia Medica of Ayurveda*

Based on Madanapala's Nighantu (New Delhi: B. Jain, 1991), 11. The fully mature leaves contain 16.74 percent protein as well as 20 mg of vitamin C in every 10 grams of leaves; see S. K. P. Sinha and J. V. V. Dogra, "Variations in the Level of Vitamin C, Total Phenolics and Protein in *Phyllanthus niruri* Linn. During Leaf Maturation," *National Academy of Science Letters* (India) 4 (1981): 467-69.

219. P. S. Venkateswaran et al., "Effects of an Extract from *Phyllanthus niruri* on Hepatitis B and Woodchick Hepatitis Viruses: *In vitro* and *in vivo* Studies," *Proceedings of the National Academy of Sciences* 84 (1987): 274–78.

220. G. V. Satyavati, "Use of Plant Drugs in Indian Traditional Systems of Medicine and Their Relevance to Primary Health Care" in *Economic and Medicinal Plant Research*, eds., H. Wagner and N. R. Farnsworth (London: Academic Press, 1990), 39–56.

221. C.-C. Hsieh et al., "Age at First Establishment of Chronic Hepatitis B Virus Infection and Hepatocellular Carcinoma Risk," *American Journal of Epidemiology* 136 (1992): 1115–21.

222. Y. Ghendon, "WHO Strategy for the Global Elimination of New Cases of Hepatitis B," *Vaccine* 8, Suppl. (1990): S129–33.

223. B. S. Blumberg et al., "Hepatitis B Virus and Primary Hepatocellular Carcinoma: Treatment of HBV Carriers with *Phyllanthus amarus*," *Vaccine* 8, Suppl. (1990): S86–92. See also note 208 above.

224. S. P. Thyagarajan et al., "*Phyllanthus amarus* and Hepatitis B," *The Lancet* 336 (October 13, 1990): 949–50.

225. Gabriel Canihuante, "Brazil: Wild Plant May Be Cure for Hepatitis B," *Inter Press Service*, December 18, 1991.

226. O. H. Fay, "Hepatitis B in Latin America: Epidemiological Patterns and Eradication Strategy," *Vaccine* 8, Suppl. (1990): S100–6.

227. Robert Cooke, "Controlling Hepatitis and Liver Cancer," *Newsday*, March 29, 1988: 3.

228. See note 223 above.

229. See note 227 above.

230. A. Leelarasamee et al., "Failure of *Phyllanthus amarus* to Eradicate Hepatitis B Surface Antigen from Symptomless Carriers," *The Lancet* 335 (June 30, 1990): 1600–1.

231. S. P. Thyagarajan et al., "Effect of *Phyllanthus amarus* on Chronic Carriers of Hepatitis B Virus," *The Lancet* 2 (October 1, 1988): 764–66.

232. B. N. Dhawan et al., "*Ex vivo* Hepatoprotective Activity of Medicinal Plants on Rat Hepatocytes," *European Journal of Pharmacology* 183 (1990): 606–7.

233. S.-F. Yeh et al., "Effect of an Extract from *Phyllanthus amarus* on Hepatitis B Surface Antigen Gene Expression in Human Hepatoma Cells," *Antiviral Research* 20 (1993): 185–92.

234. A. Munshi et al., "Evaluation of *Phyllanthus amarus* and *Phyllanthus maderaspatensis* as Agents for Postexposure Prophylaxis in Neonatal Duck Hepatitis B Virus Infection," *Journal of Medicinal Virology* 40 (1993): 53–58. See also A. Milne et al., "Failure of New Zealand Hepatitis B Carriers to Respond to *Phyllanthus amanus*," *New Zealand Medical Journal* (June 22, 1994): 243.

235. See notes 225 and 231 above.

236. M. I. Thabrew et al., "Immunomodulatory Activity of Three Sri-Lankan Medicinal Plants Used in Hepatic Disorders," *Journal of Ethnopharmacology* 33 (1991): 63–66.

237. D. W. Unander et al., "Inhibicion De La ADN Polimerasa Viral Dependiente De Virus Hepatitis B Por Especies De *Phyllanthus*, Efectos Geneticos y Ambientales Sobre Esta Actividad," *Brenesia* 34 (1991): 27–40.
238. D. W. Unander, "Callus Induction in *Phyllanthus* Species and Inhibition of Viral DNA Polymerase and Reverse Transcriptase by Callus Extracts," *Plant Cell Reports* 10 (1991): 461–66.
239. Maxwell, *Witch Doctor's Apprentice*, 372, 390.
240. "NIH Consensus Conference: Gallstones and Laparoscopic Cholecystectomy," *Journal of the American Medical Association* 269 (1993): 1018–24.
241. L. E. Luna, "The Healing Practices of a Peruvian Shaman," *Journal of Ethnopharmacology* 11 (1984): 123–33.
242. Dennis J. McKeena, Ph.D., then at the Department of Botany, University of British Columbia; personal communication, July 1983.
243. See note 241 above. In reference to Brazilian *T. incana*, see note 146 above.
244. See note 242 above.
245. Dennis J. McKeena, "Psychedelic Healing: A Proposal for a Multidisciplinary Biomedical Investigation of the Role of *Ayahuasca* in Mestizo Folk Medicine," Department of Botany, University of British Columbia, Vancouver, B.C., 1984, 17. Note that ayahuasca isn't some mildly acting recreational drug but a potent hallucinogen and a monoamine-oxidase (MAO) inhibitor that could conceivably cause neurologic impairment. That it appears to be well tolerated by the initiated remains to be studied biomedically.
246. "Harmine." In *Martindale's: The Extra Pharmacopoeia*, 28th ed. James E. F. Reynolds, ed. (London: Pharmaceutical Press, 1982), 925.
247. L. Rivier and J.-E. Lindgren, "Ayahuasca, the South American Hallucinogenic Drink: An Ethnobotanical and Chemical Investigation," *Economic Botany* 26 (1972): 101–29.
248. Kevin Krajick, "Vision Quest," *Newsweek*, June 15, 1992, 62–63.
249. See notes 241 and 242 above.
250. Luis Eduardo Luna, Swedish School of Economics, Helsinki; letter to the author, April 27, 1983.
251. Ibid.
252. V. de Feo, "Medicinal and Magical Plants in the Northern Peruvian Andes," *Fitoterapia* 63 (1992): 417-40.
253. Luis Eduardo Luna; letter to the author, September 15, 1983.
254. Maxwell, *Witch Doctor's Apprentice,* 379-80.
255. Ibid., 363–64.
256. Ibid.
257. Ibid.
258. Luis Eduardo Luna, "The Concept of Plants As Teachers Among Four Mestizo Shamans of Iquitos, Northeast Peru," paper presented at the Symposium on Shamanism, XIth International Congress of Anthropological and Ethnological Sciences, Vancouver, B.C., August 20–23, 1984, App. A: 18. See also Luis Eduardo Luna, "Vegetalismo. Shamanism Among the Mestizo Population of the Peruvian Amazon." *Acta Universitatis Stockholmiensis* 27 (1986): 202. A 1982 film by Dr. Luna, *Don Emilio and His Little Doctors*, documents the communication by an ayahuasquero with the spirit world of plants for instruction in the treatment of disease. Film inquiries can be made to Dr. Luna at the Swedish School of Economics, Arkadiankstu 22, 001000 Helsinki 10, Finland.

259. Julio Bartolo, "*Ervas medicinais* a Saude Esta Nas Plantas," *Manchete* (Rio de Janeiro), October 2, 1982: 111–15. Translation.

260. Seizi Oga, Ph.D., University of São Paulo; letter to the author, April 13, 1984.

261. Uphof, *Dictionary*, 334.

262. R. J. Spjut and R .E. Perdue, Jr., "Plant Folklore: A Tool for Predicting Sources of Antitumor Activity?" *Cancer Treatment Reports* 60 (1976): 979–85.

263. S. M. Seiber et al., "Pharmacology of Antitumor Agents from Higher Plants," *Cancer Treatment Reports* 60 (1976): 1127–39.

264. M. K. Wolpert-Defillipes et al., "Initial Studies on the Cytotoxic Action of Maytansine, a Novel Ansa Macrolide," *Biochemical Pharmacology* 24 (1975): 751–54.

265. F. Cabanillas et al., "Phase I Study of Maytansine Using a 3-Day Schedule," *Cancer Treatment Reports* 60 (1978): 429–33.

266. B. A. Chabner et al., "Initial Clinical Trials of Maytansine, an Antitumor Plant Alkaloid," *Cancer Treatment Reports* 62 (1978): 429–33.

267. M. J. O'Connell et al., "Phase II Trial of Maytansine in Patients with Advanced Colorectal Carcinoma," *Cancer Treatment Reports* 62 (1978): 1237–38.

268. M. J. Suffness and J. Douros, "Current Status of the NCI Plant and Animal Product Program," *Journal of Natural Products* 45 (1982): 1–14.

269. See notes 265 and 267 above.

270. See note 265 above.

271. A. M. Melo et al., "Primeiras Observações Do Uso Tópico Da Primina, Plumbagin E Maitenina Em Pacientes Portadores De Câncer De Pele," *Revista de Instituto de Antibióticos* (Recife) 14 (1974): 9–16.

272. O. G. de Lima et al., "Substâncias Antimicrobianas De Plantas Superiores. Comunicação XXXI. Maitenina, Nôvo Antimicrobiano com Açâo Antineoplásica, Isolade de Celastrácea de Pernambuco," *Revista do Instituto de Antibióticos* (Recife) 9 (1969): 17–25.

273. F. D. Monache et al., "Maitenin: A New Antitumoral Substance from *Maytenus* sp.," *Gazetta Chimica Italiana* 102 (1972): 317–20.

274. F. D. Monache et al., "Polpunonic Acid, a New Triterpenic Acid with Friedelane Carbon Skeleton," *Gazetta Chimica Italiana* 102 (1972): 636–46.

275. See note 271 above.

276. C. F. de Santana et al., "Primeiras Observações Sobre O Emprego Da Maitenina Em Pacientes Cancerosos," *Revista do Instituto de Antibióticos* (Recife) 11 (1971): 37–49.

277. J. L. Hartwell, "Plants Used Against Cancer: A Survey," *Lloydia* 31 (1968): 114.

278. Paul Martinez Crovetto, *Las Plantas Utilizadas en Medicina Popular en el Noroeste de Corrientes (Republica Argentina)*, Miscelanea no. 69. (Tucuman, Argentina: Ministeris de Cultura y Educacion, Foundacion Miguel Lillo, 1981), 69. Translation.

279. J. G. Gonzalez et al., "Chuchuhuasha—A Drug Used in Folk Medicine in the Amazonian and Andean Areas. A Chemical Study of *Maytenus laevis*," *Journal of Ethnopharmacology* 5 (1982): 73–77.

280. See note 278 above.

281. R. E. Dimayuga and J. Agundez, "Traditional Medicine of Baja California Sur (Mexico) I.," *Journal of Ethnopharmacology* 14 (1986): 183–93.

282. Schultes and Raffauf, *Healing Forest*, 127.

283. Ibid.

284. R. J. Marles, *The Ethnopharmacology of the Lowland Quichua of Eastern Ecuador* (doctoral thesis, University of Illinois at Chicago, 1988. Ann Arbor, Mich: University Microfilms International, 1992): 37–38.

285. F. W. Freise, "Plantas Medicinais Brasileiras," *Boletim de Agricultura* 34 (1933): 410. In Uruguay, *M. ilicifolia* is used as an external antiseptic and for asthma; see A. Gozalez et al., "Biological Screening of Uruguayan Medicinal Plants," *Journal of Ethnopharmacology* 39 (1993): 217–20.

286. See note 277 above.

287. See notes 259 and 260 above.

288. M. L. O. Souza-Formigoni et al., "Antiulcerogenic Effects of Two *Maytenus* Species in Laboratory Animals," *Journal of Ethnopharmacology* 34 (1991): 21–27.

289. Ibid.

290. C. B. Alice et al., "Screening of Plants Used in Brazilian Folk Medicine," *Journal of Ethnopharmacology* 35 (1991): 165–71.

291. See note 288 above.

292. See note 285 above.

293. M. G. M. Oliveira et al., "Pharmacologic and Toxicologic Effects of Two *Maytenus* Species in Laboratory Animals," *Journal of Ethnopharmacology* 34 (1991): 29–41.

294. P. Arenas and R. M. Azorero, "Plants Used As Means of Abortion, Contraception, Sterilization and Fecundation by Paraguayan Indigenous People," *Economic Botany* 31 (1977): 302–6.

295. P. Arenas and R. M. Azorero, "Plants of Common Use in Paraguayan Folk Medicine for Regulating Fertility," *Economic Botany* 31 (1977): 298–301.

296. See note 293 above.

297. See note 261 above.

CHAPTER FOUR

1. Valter Accorsi, University of São Paulo; letter to the author, May 27, 1983.

2. L. P. Cavalcanti, "Ipés—Bignoniaceas," *Revista Brasileira de Farmacia* 43 (1967): 141–45. Translation.

3. Jônio de Freitas Mota and Manoel Motta, "A Verdade Sobre O Ipé-Roxo," *O'Cruzeiro* (São Paulo), June 10, 1967, 6–13. Translation.

4. M. M. de Oliveira et al., "Testes Farmacológicos Iniciais com Extratos Bruto e Semipurificados de Ipê Roxo," *Arquivos do Instituto Biologico* 37, suppl. 1 (1970): 40–42. Translation. The alkaloids of *Tabebuia* remain to be elucidated.

5. E. D. Harris, "Hydrochloroquine Is Safe and Probably Useful in Rheumatoid Arthritis," *Annals of Internal Medicine* 119 (1993): 1146–47.

6. S. Oga and T. Sekino, "Toxicidade e Actividade Anti-inflamatória de *Tabebuia avellanedae* Lorentz e Griesebach (Ipê Roxo)," *Revista da Universidade de São Paulo* 7 (1969): 47-53. Translation. Note that in the text I have replaced all species given as species of *Tabebuia* and *Tecoma* with correct names following the work of Gentry (see note 55 below).

7. G. A. Nowak, *Special Active Agents and Adjuvants in Cosmetics,* vol. 1, trans., Philip Alexander (Augsburg, Germany: Verlag für Chemisch Industrie, 1985), 256.

8. J. C. Th. Uphof, *Dictionary of Economic Plants,* 2nd ed. (New York: Verlag von J. Cramer, 1968), 441.

9.   W. J. Freeland et al., "Tannins and Saponin: Interaction in Herbivore Diets," *Biochemical Systematics and Ecology* 13 (1985): 189–93.
10. See note 6 above.
11. N. Yata and O. Tanaka, "The Effects of Saponins in Promoting the Solubility and Absorption of Drugs," *Oriental Healing Arts International Bulletin* 13 (1988): 13–22.
12. O. W. Longo, "Sobre a Ocurrencia de Estroncio em Plantas do Genero *Tecoma* (Bignoniaceae)," *Academia Brasileira de Ciencias* (Rio de Janeiro) 9 (1967): 241–43. Translation.
13. C. F. de Santana et al., "Observaçoes Sobre as Propriedades ant Tumorais e Toxicológicas do Extrato d Lier e de Alguns Componentes de Cerne d Pau d'Arco *(Tabebuia avellanedae),*" *Revista do Instituto de Antibióticos* 8 (1968): 89–94. Translation.
14. N. Sharapin et al., "Triagem Anticancerigena Preliminar de Plantas Brasileiras— Part I," *Revista Brasileira de Farmacia* (January/April 1975): 19–28. Translation.
15. Otto R. Gottlieb, Institute of Chemistry, São Paulo; letter to the author, August 7, 1983.
16. "Ask the Lawrence Review," *The Lawrence Review of Natural Products* 4, no. 9 (1983): 39.
17. Jônio de Freitas Mota and Manoel Motta, "A Conspiraçao do Silêncio," *O'Cruzeiro* (São Paulo), March 25, 1967. Translation.
18. "Cancer: se cura con te¿" *Ultima Linea* (San Miguel de Tucuman, Argentina) 1, no. 12 (October 1967): 10–12. Translation.
19. Teodoro Meyer, "Nuestro Aporte: Elixer Lapachol Meyer," San Miguel de Tucuman, Tucuman Argentina, 1971. Translation.
20. H. Wagner and A. Proksch, "Immunostimulatory Drugs of Fungi and Higher Plants," in *Economic and Medicinal Plant Research,* vol. 1, eds., H. Wagner et al. (London: Academic Press, 1985), 113–53.
21. See note 19 above.
22. W.-Y. Li and E. J. Lien, "Fu-zhen Herbs in the Treatment of Cancer," *Oriental Healing Arts International Bulletin* 11 (1986): 1–8.
23. F. J. DiCarlo et al., "Reticuloendothelial System Stimulants of Botanical Origin," *Journal of the Reticuloendothelial Society* 1 (1964): 224–32.
24. Ibid.
25. S. J. Record and R. W. Hess, "American Timbers of the Family Bignoniaceae," *Tropical Woods*, no. 63 (1949): 9–38.
26. Ibid.
27. Hernando Garcia Barriga, *Flora Medicinal De Colombia. Botanica Medica* (Bogota, Colombia: Instituto de Ciencias Naturales, Universidad Nacional, 1975), 143–48. Translation.
28. Richard Evans Schultes and Robert F. Raffauf, *The Healing Forest: Medicinal and Toxic Plants of the Northwest Amazonia* (Portland, Ore.: Dioscorides Press, 1990), 107–8.
29. L. C. Branch and M. F. da Silva, "Folk Medicine of Alter Do Chão, Pará, Brazil," *Acta Amazonica* 13 (1983): 737–97.
30. See note 23 above.
31. Ibid.
32. Y. Hokama, University of Hawaii at Manoa; personal communication, April 1985.

33. Ibid.
34. Ibid.
35. S. A. Y. Suzuki et al., "Low Dalton Non-Polar Compounds from Extracts of *Tecoma conspicua* Bark with Antitumor Activity and Potential Immuno-modulator Activity," *Federation Proceedings* 44 (1985): 912.
36. T. A. Sprague and N. Y. Sandwith, "Contributions to the Flora of Tropical America: IX.," *Bulletin of Miscellaneous Information,* Royal Botanic Gardens, Kew, London (1932): 18–28.
37. Stephany Grozdea (Rio de Janeiro); personal communication, May 1983.
38. See note 35 above.
39. David H. Moikeha, Jr., and Y. Hokama, "Effect of Crude *Tabebuia* Extracts *in Vitro* and *in Vivo* on Macrophages and Lewis Lung Carcinoma in C57B1/6J Mice." (Department of Pathology, John A. Burns School of Medicine, University of Hawaii, Honolulu, Hawaii, 1986, unpublished), 21 pp.
40. Kenneth Corwin, Santa Monica, California; personal communication, April 1985.
41. See note 39 above.
42. Ibid.
43. Ibid.
44. Dr. Hildebert Wagner, University of Munich; personal communication, July 1987.
45. Dr. Hildebert Wagner; personal communication, May 1986.
46. Dr. Hildebert Wagner; letter to the author, August 25, 1986.
47. See note 45 above.
48. See notes 13 and 14 above.
49. B. J. Abbott et al., "Screening Data from the Cancer Chemotherapy National Service Center Screening Laboratories. XXXII. Plant Extracts," *Cancer Research* 26, suppl., part 2 (1966): 417.
50. B. J. Abbott et al., "Screening Data from the Cancer Chemotherapy National Service Center Screening Laboratories. XL. Plant Extracts," *Cancer Research* 27, suppl., part 2 (1966): 326.
51. J. Leiter et al., "Screening Data from the Cancer Chemotherapy National Service Center Screening Laboratories. IX. Plant Extracts," *Cancer Research* 22, suppl., part 2 (1962): 647, 677, 693.
52. B. J. Abbott et al., "Screening Data from the Cancer Chemotherapy National Service Center Screening Laboratories. XXXVIII. Plant Extracts," *Cancer Research* 26, suppl., part 2 (1966): 1478.
53. J. Leiter et al., "Screening Data from the Cancer Chemotherapy National Service Center Screening Laboratories. VI. Plant Extracts," *Cancer Research* 21, part 2 (1961): 106, 146.
54. B. J. Abbott et al., "Screening Data from the Cancer Chemotherapy National Service Center Screening Laboratories. XXXIV. Plant Extracts," *Cancer Research* 26, suppl., part 2 (1966): 796, 888.
55. Alwyn H. Gentry, *Bignoniaceae—Part II (Tecomeae). Flora Neotropica*, Monograph 25, no. 11 (New York: New York Botanical Garden, 1992), 251–52.
56. See note 51 above.
57. See notes 49–54 above.
58. See notes 39 and 45 above.
59. A. F. Brodie, "Naphthoquinones in Oxidative Metabolism," in *Biochemistry*

of Quinones, ed., R. A. Morton (London: Academic Press, 1965), 355–59.

60. E. Cadenas and P. Hochstein, "Pro- and Antioxidant Functions of Quinones and Quinone Reductases in Mammalian Cells," *Advances in Enzymology* 65 (1992): 97–146.

61. J. Segura-Aguillar and C. Lind, "On the Mechanism of the Mn^{+3}-induced Neurotoxicity of Dopamine: Prevention of Quinone-Derived Oxygen Toxicity by DT Diaphorase and Superoxide Dismutase," *Chemico-Biological Interactions* 72 (1989): 309–24.

62. R. E. Beyer et al., "Evaluation of Tissue Coenzyme Q (Ubiquinone) and Cytochrome c Concentrations by Endurance Exercise in the Rat," *Archives of Biochemistry and Biophysics* 234 (1984): 323–29.

63. K. Okamoto et al., "Synthesis of Quinones Having Carboxy- and Hydroxy-Alkyl Side Chains, and Their Effects on Rat-Liver Lysosomal Membrane," *Chemical and Pharmaceutical Bulletin* 30 (1982): 2797–2819.

64. Bill Lawren, "A New Piece in the Aging Puzzle," *Longevity* magazine (July 1990): 35–37.

65. M. Lingetti et al., "Evaluation of the Clinical Efficacy of Idebenone in Patients Affected by Chronic Cerebrovascular Disorders," *Archives of Gerontology* 15 (1992): 225–37.

66. V. Senin et al., "Idebenone in Senile Dementia of Alzheimer Type: A Multicentre Study," *Archives of Gerontology and Geriatrics* 15 (1992): 249–60.

67. B. Bergamasco et al., "Effects of Idebenone in Elderly Subjects with Cognitive Decline. Results of a Multicentre Clinical Trial," *Archives of Gerontology and Geriatrics* 15 (1992): 279–86.

68. G. Nappi et al., "Long-Term Idebenone Treatment of Vascular and Degenerative Brain Disorders of the Elderly," *Archives of Gerontology and Geriatrics* 15 (1992): 261–69.

69. See note 66 above.

70. See note 64 above.

71. Harold A. Harper et al., *Review of Physiological Chemistry*, 16th ed. (Los Altos, Calif.: Lange Medical Publications, 1977), 152–54.

72. A. R. Burnett and R. H. Thompson, "Naturally Occurring Quinones. Part X. The Quinonoid Constituents of *Tabebuia avellanedae* (Bignoniaceae)," *Journal of the Chemical Society*, part C (1967): 2100–4.

73. R. E. Talcott et al., "Inhibition of Microsomal Lipid Peroxidation by Naphthoquinones: Structure-Activity Relationships and Possible Mechanisms of Action," *Archives of Biochemistry and Biophysics* 241 (1985): 88-94.

74. See note 63 above.

75. L. H. Block et al., "Nonspecific Resistance to Bacterial Infections: Enhancement by Ubiquinone-8," *Journal of Experimental Medicine* 148 (1978): 1228–40.

76. I. Azuma, "Effect of Ubiquinones and Related Compounds on Immune Responses in Mice and Guinea Pigs," *Vitamins* (Japan) 52 (1978): 503–7.

77. I. Azuma et al., "The Effect of Ubiquinone-7 and Its Metabolites on the Immune Response," *International Journal of Vitamin and Nutrition Research* 48 (1978): 255–61.

78. K. Folkers et al., "Biochemical Rationale and the Cardiac Response of Patients with Muscle Disease to Therapy with Coenzyme Q10," *Proceedings of the National Academy of Sciences* 82 (1985): 4513.

79. J. Tanaka et al., "Coenzyme Q10: The Prophylactic Effect on Low Cardiac

Output Following Cardiac Valve Replacement," *Annals of Thoracic Surgery* 33 (1982): 145.

80. K. Folkers et al., "Bioenergetics in Clinical Medicine—X. Survey of the Adjunctive Use of Coenzyme Q with Oral Therapy in Treating Peridontal Disease," *Journal of Medicine* 8 (1977): 333–48.

81. Kenneth Anderson and Lois Anderson, *Orphan Drugs* (Los Angeles, Calif.: The Body Press, 1987), 206.

82. E. G. Bliznakov et al., "Coenzyme Q Deficiency in Aged Mice," *Journal of Medicine* 9 (1978): 337.

83. E. G. Bliznakov, "Immunological Senescence in Mice and Its Reversal by Coenzyme Q10," *Mechanisms of Aging Development* 7 (1978): 189.

84. E. G. Bliznakov and G. L. Hunt, *The Miracle Nutrient Coenzyme Q10* (New York: Bantam Books, 1987), 28–29.

85. G. Proserpio, "Natural Sunscreens: Vegetable Derivatives as Sunscreens and Tanning Agents," *Cosmetics and Toiletries* 91 (March 1976): 34–46.

86. R. M. Fusaro et al., "Sunlight Protection in Normal Skin," *Archives of Dermatology* 93 (1966): 106–11.

87. R. H. Thompson, *Naturally Occurring Quinones.* (London and New York: Academic Press, 1971).

88. H.-Y. Hsu et al., "Physiologically Active Constituents of Red Sage (*Salvia miltorrhiza* Bunge)," *Oriental Healing Arts International Bulletin* 12 (1987): 422–28.

89. X. Peigen, "Recent Developments on Medicinal Plants in China," *Journal of Ethnopharmacology* 7 (1983): 95–109.

90. A. R. Burnett and R. H. Thompson, "Naturally Occurring Quinones. Part XII. Extractives from *Tabebuia chrysantha* Nichols and Other Bignoniaceae," *Journal of the Chemical Society*, part C (1968): 850–53.

91. See note 72 above.

92. J. Sterlz et al., "The Immuno-Inhibitory and Immunostimulatory Effects of Hydroxyanthra—and Hydroxynaphthoquinone Derivatives," *Folia Microbiologica* 26 (1981): 169–75.

93. H. Wagner et al., "Immunological Investigations of Naphthoquinone-Containing Plant Extracts, Isolated Quinones and Other Cytostatic Compounds in Cellular Immunosystems," *Planta Medica*,no. 6 (1986): 550. Poster.

94. H. Wagner et al., "*In Vitro* Stimulation of Human Granulocytes and Lymphocytes by Pico- and Femtogram Quantities of Cytostatic Agents," *Arzneimittel-Forschung* (Drug Research) 38 (1988): 273–76.

95. See note 46 above.

96. Bernhard Kreher, *Chemische und Immunologische Untersuchungen der Drogen Dionaea muscipula, Tabebuia avellanedae, Euphorbia resinifera und Daphne mezereum Sowie Iher Präparate* (dissertation of the faculty of Chemistry and Pharmacy of Ludwig-Maximilians University, Munich, June 1989), 37–89, 160–62. Translation.

97. See note 93 above.

98. See note 94 above.

99. H. Wagner, "Leading Structures of Plant Origin for Drug Development," *Journal of Ethnopharmacology* 38 (1993): 105–12.

100. See note 94 above.

101. Carnivora-Deutschland GmbH. *Dionaea Muscipula Venus-Fliegenfalle.* Jagsthausen, West Germany, 1983, 9 pp.

102. "Venusfliegenfalle hilft nicht," *Arztliche Praxis* 37 (1985): 3150.
103. "Phytotheraputika in der Krebsbehandlung: Ultima ration oder Mittel der Wahl?," *Apotheker Journal* S (1985): 44.
104. See notes 93 and 96 above.
105. B. Kreher et al., "New Furanonaphthoquinones and Other Constituents of *Tabebuia avellanedae* and Their Immunomodulating Activities *in Vitro*," *Planta Medica* 54, no. 6 (1988): 562. Poster.
106. See note 93 above.
107. Samuel J. Record and Clayton D. Mell. *Timbers of Tropical America* (New Haven, Conn.: Yale University Press, 1924), 530–33.
108. O. G. de Lima et al., "Uma Nova Substancia Antibiótica Isolada do 'Pau d'Arco,' *Tabebuia* sp.," *Anais da Sociedade de Biologia de Pernambuco* 14 (1956): 136–40. Translation.
109. M. L. S. Linhares and C. F. de Santana, "Estudo Sobre o Efeito de Substâncias Antibióticas Obtidas de Stretomyces e Vegetais Superiores Sobre o *Herpesvirus hominis*," *Revista do Instituto de Antibióticos* (Recife) 15 (1975): 25–32. Translation.
110. M. H. do C. Lagrota et al., "Atividade Antiviróica Do Lapachol," *Revista De Microbiologica* (São Paulo) 14 (1983): 21–26. Translation.
111. R. K. Goel et al., "Effect of Lapachol, a Naphthoquinone Isolated from *Tectona grandis*, on Experimental Peptic Ulcer and Gastric Secretion," *Journal of Pharmacy and Pharmacology* 39 (1987): 138–40.
112. E. R. de Almeida et al., "Antiinflammatory Action of Lapachol," *Journal of Ethnopharmacology* 29 (1990): 239–41.
113. K. Kinoshita et al., "Inhibitory Effects of Plant Secondary Metabolites on Cytotoxic Activity of Polymorphonuclear Leucocytes," *Planta Medica* 58 (1992): 137–45.
114. See note 112 above.
115. E. R. dos Santos et al., "Estudos de difusão cutânea do lapachol I—Ensaios (*in vitro*)," *Revista Portuguesa de Farmacia* 41 (1991): 15–19.
116. Laboratório Farmaceutico do Estado de Pernambuco S.A. *LAFEPE*, 1982, Recife, Brazil. Product brochure.
117. S. K. Carter et al., "Lapachol—NSC 11905—Clinical Brochure." National Cancer Institute (Chemotherapy), November 1967, 13 pp.
118. Oswaldo G. de Lima, Institute of Antibiotics, Recife, Brazil; personal communication, May 1983. See also note 112.
119. C. F. de Santana et al., "Primeiras Observaçoes com Emprego do Lapachol em Pacientes Humanos Portadores de Neoplasias Malignas," *Revista do Instituto de Antibioticos* 20 (1980/1): 61–68.
120. Ibid.
121. M. Suffness and J. Douros, "Current Status of the NCI Plant and Animal Product Program," *Journal of Natural Products* 45 (1982): 1–14.
122. J. B. Block et al., "Early Clinical Studies with Lapachol (NSC—11905)," *Cancer Chemotherapy Reports* 4, no. 4, part 2 (1974): 27–28.
123. K. V. Rao et al., "Recognition and Evaluation of Lapachol As an Antitumor Agent," *Cancer Research* 28 (1968): 1952–54.
124. See note 121 above.
125. See note 119 above.
126. C. Y. Lui et al., "Some Formulation Properties of Lapachol, a Potential Oncolytic

Agent of Natural Origin," *Drug Development and Industrial Pharmacy* 11 (1985): 1763–79. Pharmacologists C.Y. Lui and colleagues of the College of Pharmacy at the University of Illinois at Chicago found that alkaline (buffered) water enormously increased the solubility of lapachol. With a dilution of lapachol with buffered water at a pH of 7.4, which is physiological pH, or the pH of our bodies, the problem that the NCI encountered of not being able to inject lapachol because of precipitation into its coarse, crystalline form when diluted with water, seems close to being solved: lapachol stayed in solution. Soybean oil improved solubility six times more than water (pH 8.0). Further research might turn up even better vehicles.

127. E. R. de Almeida et al., "The Action of 2-Hydroxy-3-(3-Methyl-2-Butenyl)-1,4-naphthoquinone (Lapachol) in Pregnant Rats," *Revista Portuguesa de Farmacia* 38 (1988): 21–23.
128. See note 123 above.
129. J. L. Hartwell, "Plants Used Against Cancer: A Survey," *Journal of Natural Products* 31 (1968): 76.
130. K. C. Joshi et al., "Chemical Examination of the Roots of *Stereospermum suaveolens* D.C.," *Journal of the Indian Chemical Society* 54 (1977): 648–49.
131. Vaidya Radhika and A. V. Balasubramanian, *Mother and Child Care in Traditional Medicine: Part I*, LSPP Monograph no. 3 (Madras, India: P.P.S.T. Foundation, 1990), 48–49.
132. N. G. Patel, "Ayurveda: The Traditional Medicine of India," in *Folk Medicine: The Art and the Science*, ed., Richard P. Steiner (Washington, D.C.: American Chemical Society, 1986), 41–65.
133. See note 1 above.
134. Valter Accorsi, University of São Paulo; personal communication, May 1983.
135. Fadlo Fraige Filho, São Paulo; personal communication, June 1983.
136. Milan Dimitri and Jose Biloni, *El Libro Del Arbol* (Buenos Aires: Celulosa Argentina, 1973). Translation.
137. See note 13 above.
138. See note 1 above.
139. See note 135 above.
140. K. H. Schulz et al., "The Sensitizing Capacity of Naturally Occurring Quinones—Experimental Studies in Guinea Pigs," *Archives for Dermatological Research* 258 (1977): 41–52.
141. Etain Cronin, *Contact Dermatitis* (New York: Churchill Livingston 1980), 556.
142. H. K. Krogh, "Contact Eczema Caused by True Teak," *British Journal of Industrial Medicine* 21 (1964): 65–68.
143. See note 1 above.
144. See note 142 above.
145. See note 135 above.
146. M. C. Wanick et al., "Acao Antiinflamatória e Cicatrizante do Extrato Hidroalcoólico do Liber do Pau d'Arco Roxo (*Tabebuia avellanedae*), em Pacientes Portadores de Cervicites e Cérvico-Vaginites," *Seperata da Revista do Instituto de Antibiotics* 10 (1970): 41–46.
147. Ibid.
148. E. J. Van Stott and R. H. Bonder, "Intravaginal and Intrarectal Screening of Antimitotic Drugs for Topical Effectiveness," *Journal of Investigative Dermatology* 50 (1971): 132–39.

149. P. H. List and L. Horhammer, *Hagers Handbuch der Pharmazeutischen Praxis* 60, part C, 4th ed. (Berlin: Springer-Verlag, 1979), 29.

150. See note 112 above.

151. O. G. de Lima et al., "Substâncias Antimicrobianas de Plantas Superiores. Comunicação XX. Atividade Antimicrobiana de Alguns Derivados do Lapachol em Comparação com a Xiloidona, Nova Orto-Naftoquinona Natural Isolada de Extratos do Cerne do 'Pau d'Arco' Rôxo, *Tabebuia avellanedae* Lor. ex Griseb," *Revista do Instituto de Antibióticos* (Recife) 4 (1962): 3–17. See also P. Guiraud et al., "Comparison of Antibacterial and Antifungal Activities of Lapachol and β-Lapachone," *Planta Medica* 60 (1994):373–74.

152. O. G. de Lima et al., "Substâncias Antimicrobianas de Plantas Superiores. Comunicação XXXV. Atividade Antimicrobiana e Antitumoral de Lawsona (2-hidroxi-1,4-naftoquinona) em Comparação com o Lapachol (2-hidroxi-3-(-3-metil-2-butenil)-1,4-naftoquinona)," *Revista do Instituto de Antibióticos* (Recife) 11 (1971): 21–27.

153. See note 72 above.

154. See note 149 above.

155. W. E. Flood, *Dictionary of Chemical Names* (Totawa, N.J.: Littlefield, Adams, 1967), 195, 48. Aspirin taken orally has shown good results in the treatment of chronic venous ulcers of the legs, but why this is so has still to be worked out. See A. M. Layton, et al., "Randomised Trial of Oral Aspirin for Chronic Venous Leg Ulcers," *The Lancet* 344 (July 16, 1994): 164–65.

156. "Benzoic acid" and "*p*-hydroxybenzoic acid" in *Dorland's Illustrated Medical Dictionary*, 26th ed. (Philadelphia: W. B. Saunders, 1981), 14, 17.

157. M. Fukushima and S. Kimura, "Studies on Cosmetic Ingredients from Crude Drugs (I). Inhibition of Tyrosinase Activity by Crude Drugs," *Shoyakugaku Zasshi* 43 (1989): 142–47.

158. P. A. Riley, "The Mechanism of Skin Pigmentation," *Journal of the Society of Cosmetic Chemists* 28 (1977): 395–401.

159. M. A. Pathak and K. Stratton, "Free Radicals in Human Skin Before and After Exposure to Light," *Archives of Biochemistry and Biophysics* 123 (1968): 468–76.

160. L. M. Edelstein, "Melanin: A Unique Biopolymer," *Pathology Annual* 1 (1971): 309–24.

161. F. E. Barr et al., "Melanin: The Organizing Molecule," *Medical Hypotheses* 11 (1983): 39–40.

162. See note 157 above.

163. Walter Lewis and Memory P. F. Elvin-Lewis, *Medical Botany* (New York: John Wiley, 1977), 343.

164. See note 155 above.

165. "Benzoic acid" in *Kirk-Othmer Encyclopedia of Chemical Technology*, vol. 3, 3rd ed. (New York: John Wiley, 1981), 778–92.

166. "Benzoic Acid" in *Martindale. The Extra Pharmacopoeia*, 29th ed. J. E. F. Reynolds, ed. (London: Pharmaceutical Press, 1989), 1355-56.

167. See note 165 above.

168. Editorial. "The Natural Way Ahead?" *Manufacturing Chemist* 60 (1989): 33, 40.

169. R. B. Aronsohn, "Skin Treating Formulation," *Chemical Abstracts* 105 (1986): 361, C.A. 105: 158638k.

170. See note 96 above.

171. M. Satyavathi et al., "Chemosystematics of *Tabebuia*," *Korean Journal of Botany* 33 (1990): 55–58.
172. B. Havsteen, "Flavonoids, a Class of Natural Products of High Pharmacological Potency," *Biochemical Pharmacology* 32 (1983): 1141–48.
173. E. Middleton et al., "Quercetin: An Inhibitor of Antigen-Induced Human Basophil Histamine Release," *Journal of Immunology* 127 (1981): 546–50.
174. G. D. Lutterodt, "Inhibition of Gastrointestinal Release of Acetylcholine by Quercetin As a Possible Mode of Action of *Psidium guajava* Leaf Extracts in the Treatment of Acute Diarrheal Disease," *Journal of Ethnopharmacology* 25 (1989): 235–47.
175. R. Hoffman et al., "Enhanced Anti-Proliferative Action of Busulphon by Quercetin on the Human Leukemia Cell Line K562," *British Journal of Cancer* 59 (1989): 347–48.
176. C. Ip and H. E. Ganther, "Combination of Blocking Agents and Suppressing Agents in Cancer Prevention," *Carcinogenesis* 12 (1991): 1193–96.
177. E. E. Deschner et al., "Quercetin and Rutin As Inhibitors of Azoxymethanol-Induced Colonic Neoplasia," *Carcinogenesis* 12 (1991): 1193–96.
178. G. Scambia et al., "Inhibitory Effect of Quercetin on OVCA 433 Cells and Presence of Type II Oestrogen Binding Sites in Primary Ovarian Tumours and Cultured Cells," *British Journal of Cancer* 62 (1990): 942–46.
179. Y. Graziani and R. Chayoth, "Elevation of Cyclic AMP Level in Ehrlich Ascites Tumor Cells by Quercetin," *Biochemical Pharmacology* 26 (1977): 1259–61.
180. E.-M. Suolinna et al., "Quercetin, an Artificial Regulator of the High Aerobic Glycolysis of Tumor Cells," *Journal of the National Cancer Institute* 53 (1974): 1515–19.
181. E. Ohnishi and H. Bannai, "Quercetin Potentiates TNF-Induced Antiviral Activity," *Antiviral Research* 22 (1993): 327–33.
182. N. Ito and I. Hirono, "Is Quercetin Carcinogenic?" *Japanese Journal of Cancer Research* 83 (1992): 312–14. See also M. G. L. Hertog, "Content of Potentially Anticarcinogenic Flavonoids of Tea Infusions, Wines, and Fruit Juices," *Journal of Agriculture and Food Chemistry* 41 (1993): 1242–46.
183. M. G. L. Hertog et al., "Intake of Potentially Anticarcinogenic Flavonoids and Their Determinants in Adults in the Netherlands," *Nutrition and Cancer* 20 (1993): 21–29.
184. S. Sankara et al., "Flavonoids of Eight Bignoniaceous Plants," *Phytochemistry* 11 (1972): 1499.
185. "Tannic acid" in *Martindale's: The Extra Pharmacopoeia*, 28th ed. James Reynolds, ed. (London: Pharmaceutical Press, 1982), 287.
186. See notes 72 and 90 above.
187. B. K. Rohatgi et al., "Quinones from *Tecoma pentaphylla*: Constitution of Tecomaquinones I and II," *Indian Journal of Chemistry* 22B, sect. B (1983): 886–89.
188. See note 13 above.
189. A. R. Schuerch and W. Wehrli, "*B*-Lapachone, an Inhibitor of Oncornavirus Reverse Transcriptase and Eukaryotic DNA Polymerase-*Alpha*," *European Journal of Biochemistry* 84 (1978): 197–205.
190. D. A. Boothman et al., "Inhibition of Potentially Lethal DNA Damage Repair in Human Tumor Cells by *B*-Lapachone, an Activator of Topoisomerase I," *Cancer Research* 49 (1989): 605–12.
191. C. J. Li et al., "Three Inhibitors of Type 1 Human Immunodeficiency Virus

Long Terminal Repeat-Directed Gene Expression and Virus Replication," *Proceedings of the National Academy of Sciences USA* 90 (1993): 1839–42.

192. H. P. T. Ammon et al., "Mechanism of Anti-Inflammatory Actions of Curcumin and Boswellic Acids," *Journal of Ethnopharmacology* 38 (1993): 113–19.

193. See note 191 above.

194. R. J. Boorstein and A. B. Pardee, "*B*-Lapachone Greatly Enhances MMS Lethality to Human Fibroblasts," *Biochemical and Biophysical Research Communications* 118 (1984): 828–34.

195. See note 190 above.

196. Y.-H. Hsiang et al., "Camptothecin Induces Protein-Linked DNA Breaks via Mammalian DNA Topoisomerase I," *Journal of Biological Chemistry* 260 (1985): 14873–78.

197. D. A. Boothman et al., "Potentiation of Halogenated Pyrimidine Radiosensitizers in Human Carcinoma Cells by *B*-Lapachone (3,4-dihydro-2,2-dimethyl-2*H*-naphthol[1,2-*b*]pyran-5,6-dione), a Novel DNA Repair Inhibitor," *Cancer Research* 47 (1987): 5361–66.

198. Christopher Joyce, "Western Medicine Men Return to the Field," *BioScience* 46 (1992): 399–403.

199. W. D. Kingsbury et al., "Synthesis of Water-Soluble (Aminoakyl) Camptothecin Analogues: Inhibition of Topoisomerase I and Antitumor Activity," *Journal of Medicinal Chemistry* 34 (1991): 98–107. See also G. J. Creemers et al., "Topoisomerase I Inhibitors: Topotecan and Irenotecan," *Cancer Treatment Reviews* 20 (1994): 93–96.

200. D. A. Boothman et al., "Anticarcinogenic Potential of DNA-Repair Modulators," *Mutation Research* 202 (1988): 393–411.

201. See note 190 above.

202. H. C. Schroeder et al., "Differential *in vitro* Anti-HIV Activity of Natural Lignans," *Zeitschrift fur Naturforschung, C: Biosciences* 45 (1990): 1215–21.

203. F. Degrassi et al., "Chromosome Damage and DNA Strand Breakage by *B*-Lapachone, an Activator of Topoisomerase I," *Mutagenesis* 7 (1992): 388.

204. A. Y. Chen et al., "Menadione (Vitamin K_3) Induces Topoisomerase II-Mediated DNA Cleavage," *Proceedings of the Eighty-Third Annual Meeting of the American Association of Cancer Research* 33 (1992): 433 (Abstract 2588).

205. See note 96 above.

206. D. V. C. Awang, "Commercial Taheebo Lacks Active Ingredient," *Canadian Pharmaceutical Journal* (May 1988): 323–26.

207. See notes 46 and 93 above.

208. See note 182 above.

209. See note 206 above.

210. Bernhard Kreher, University of Munich; letter to the author, December 16, 1987.

211. M. Girard et al., "Naphthoquinone Constituents of *Tabebuia* spp.," *Journal of Natural Products* 51 (1988): 1023–24.

212. A. H. Gentry, "The Cultivated Species of *Tabebuia* with Notes on Other Bignoniaceae," *Proceedings of the Third Menninger Flowering Tree Conference*, 1982, 52–69.

213. Gentry, *Bignoniaceae—Part II*, 163–64.

214. Ibid. and see also note 212 above.

215. M. M. Rao and D. G. I. Kingston, "Plant Anticancer Agents. XII. Isolation and Structure Elucidation of New Cytotoxic Quinones from *Tabebuia cassinoides*," *Journal of Natural Products* 45 (1982): 600–604.

216. F. W. Freise, "Plantas Medicinais Brasileiras," *Boletim de Agricultura* 34 (1933): 420–24. Translation.

217. M. Pio Correa, *Diccionario das Plantas Uteis do Brasil*. Miniterio da Agricultura, Rio de Janeiro, 1969.

218. See note 96 above.

219. H. Wagner et al., "74. Structure Determination of New Isomeric Naphtho[2,3-*b*]furan-4,9-diones from *Tabebuia avellanedae* by Selective-IEPT Technique," *Helvetica Chimica Acta* (Seperatum) 72 (1989): 659–67.

220. E. A. Moreira et al., "Análise Fitoquímica Sumária Do Cortex Do 'Ipê Roxo,'" *Tribuna Farmaceutica* 35 (1967): 23–26.

221. C. L. Zani, "Isolation and Synthesis of Furanonapthoquinones (FNQ) from *Tabebuia ochracea* Cham. (Bignoniaceae)," *Brazilian-Sino Symposium on Chemistry and Pharmacology of Natural Products*, Rio de Janeiro, December 10–14, 1989. Ministry of State, Foundation Oswaldo Cruz. Poster P144: p. 210.

222. M. O. Hamburger and G. A. Cordell, "Furanonaphthoquinones from *Tabebuia avellanedae* (Bignoniaceae)," in *International Congress on Natural Products Research*, ed. James E. Robbers. American Society of Pharmacognosy and Japanese Society of Pharmacognosy, Twenty-ninth Annual Meeting of the American Society of Pharmacognosy, Park City, Utah, July 17–21, 1988. Poster 0:50.

223. S. Ueda and H. Tokuda, "Inhibitory Effect of *Tabebuia avellanedae* Constituents on Tumor Promotion," *Planta Medica* 56 (1990): 669 (Poster).

224. Y. Fujimoto et al., "Studies on the Structure and Stereochemistry of Cytotoxic Furanonaphthoquinones from *Tabebuia impetiginosa*: 5- and 8-Hydroxy-2-(1-hydroxyethyl)naphtho[2,3-*b*]furan-4,9-diones," *Journal of the Chemical Society, Perkin Transactions* 1 (1991): 2323–27.

225. Tetsuro Ikekawa; letter to the author, November 26, 1993.

226. See note 96 above.

227. K. Inoue et al., "A Naphthoquinones and a Lignan from the Wood of *Kigelia pinnata*," *Phytochemistry* 20 (1981): 2271–76. Owing to the large sausage-like fruits that hang from the branches of this tree, *K. pinnata* is widely known as the sausage or cucumber tree. Sausage trees 70 feet tall have been found in the former Rhodesia. African tribes render the fruits into powder, which is then used to dress ulcers. See Eve Palmer and Norah Pitman, *Trees of South Africa* (Amsterdam: A.A. Balkema, 1961), 318-20.

228. S. Ueda et al., "Production of Anti–Tumor-Promoting Furanonaphthoquinones in *Tabebuia avellanedae* Cell Cultures," *Phytochemistry* 36 (1994): 323-25.

229. T. Ikegawa et al., "Furonapthoquinone Derivatives, Antitumor Agents Containing Them, and Their Isolation from *Tabebuia avellanedae*." Japanese Patent 63–196576, August 15, 1988, 5 pp. (in Japanese).

230. See note 221 above.

231. R. Ribeiro-Rodrigues et al., "Naphthofuran and Naphthofuranquinone Derivatives As Inhibitors of *Trypanosoma cruzi* Epimastigotes Growth in Culture," *Brazilian-Sino Symposium on Chemistry and Pharmacology of Natural Products*, Rio de Janeiro, December 10–14, 1989. Ministry of State, Foundation Oswaldo Cruz. Poster P143: p. 209.

232. L. H. Carvalho et al., "*In vitro* and *in vivo* Antimalarial Activities of Furannaphthoquinones Produced by Modification of an Active Chemically Defined Molecule," *Brazilian-Sino Symposium on Chemistry and Pharmacology of Natural*

Products, Rio de Janeiro, December 10–14, 1989. Poster P136: p. 202.

233. J. D. Grazziotin et al., "Phytochemical and Analgesic Investigation of *Tabebuia chrysotricha,*" *Journal of Ethnopharmacology* 38 (1993): 249–51.

234. See note 23 above.

235. D. W. Bishay et al., "Macro- and Micromorphology of *Tabebuia pentaphylla* Hemsl. Cultivated in Egypt. Part II: The Stem Bark and Flower," *Bulletin of Pharmaceutical Sciences, Assuit University* 10, part 1 (1987): 50–73.

236. D. W. Bishay et al., "Phytochemical Study of *Tabebuia pentaphylla* Hemsl. Cultivated in Egypt," *Bulletin of Pharmaceutical Sciences, Assuit University* 10, part 2 (1987): 1–20.

237. Gentry, *Bignoniaceae—Part II,* 249–51, 193–98.

238. See note 236 above.

239. I. Prakash and R. Singh, "Chemical Constituents of Stem Bark and Root Heartwood of *Tabebuia pentaphylla* (Linn.) Hemsl. (Bignoniaceae)," *Pharmazie* 35 (1980): 813.

240. K. Sheth et al., "Tumor-Inhibiting Agent from *Hyptis emoryi* (Labiatea)," *Journal of Pharmaceutical Sciences* 61 (1972): 1819.

241. Uphof, *Dictionary,* 277. See also M. Kuhnt et al., *Planta Medica* 58, suppl. 1 (1992): A643–44.

242. Richard A. Rutter, *Catalogo De Plantas Utiles De La Amazonia Peruana* (Yarinacocha, Pucallpa, Peru: Ministerio de Educacion, Instituto Lingüística de Verano, 1990), 114.

243. See note 29 above.

244. K. Yasukawa et al., "Sterol and Triterpene Derivatives from Plants Inhibit the Effects of a Tumor Promotor, and Sitosterol and Betulinic Acid Inhibit Tumor Formation in Mouse Skin Two-Stage Carcinogenesis," *Oncology* 48 (1991): 72–76.

245. See note 223 above.

246. See note 244 above.

247. Uphof, *Dictionary,* p. 284.

248. S.-M. Wong et al., "Isolation and Characterization of a New Triterpene from *Iris missouriensis,*" *Journal of Natural Products* 49 (1986): 330–33.

249. J. Kitajima et al., "Two New Triterpenoid Sulphates from the Leaves of *Schefflera octophylla,*" *Chemical and Pharmaceutical Bulletin* 38 (1990): 714–16.

250. "Betula" and "Betulin" in *The Merck Index,* 11th ed., S. Budauri et al., eds. (Rahway, N.J.: Merck and Co., 1989), 185–86.

251. See note 244 above.

252. C. N. Lin et al., "Novel Cytotoxic Principles of Formosan *Ganoderma lucidum,*" *Journal of Natural Products* 54 (1991): 998–1000.

253. T. Van Sung and G. Adam, "An Acetylated Bidesmosidic Saponin from *Schefflera octophylla,*" *Journal of Natural Products* 55 (1992): 503–5.

254. S. Saito et al., "Comparison of Cytoprotective Effects of Saponins Isolated from Leaves of *Aralia elata* Seem. (Araliaceae) with Synthesized Bisdesmosides of Oleanolic Acid and Hederagenin on Carbon Tetrachloride-Induced Hepatic Injury," *Chemical and Pharmaceutical Bulletin* 41 (1993): 1395–1401.

255. N. Basu and R. P. Rastogi, "Triterpenoid Saponins and Sapogenins," *Phytochemistry* 6 (1967): 1249–70.

256. See note 223 above.

257. See note 244 above. Taken orally by mice, oleanolic acid showed a rate of anti-inflammatory action comparable to that of glycyrrhetinic acid, a triterpene

found in licorice root. See E. Sugishita et al., "Structure-Activity Studies of Some Oleanane Triterpenoid Glycosides and Their Related Compounds from the Leaves of *Tetrapanax papyriferum* on Anti-inflammatory Activities," *Journal of Pharmacobio-Dynamics* 5 (1982): 379–87.

258. Y. Muto et al., "Present Status of Research on Cancer Chemoprevention in Japan," *Japanese Journal of Oncology* 20 (1990): 219–24. See also K.-H. Lee et al., *Planta Medica* 54 (1988): 308–11.

259. S. Balanehru and B. Nagarajan, "Protective Effect of Oleanolic Acid and Ursolic Acid Against Lipid Peroxidation," *Biochemistry International* 24 (1991): 981–90.

260. S. Balanehru and B. Nagarajan, "Intervention of Adriamycin Induced Free Radical Damage," *Biochemistry International* 28 (1992): 735–44.

261. Y. Liu et al., "Oleanolic Acid Protects against Cadmium Hepatotoxicity by Inducing Metallothionein," *Journal of Pharmacology and Experimental Therapeutics* 266 (1993): 400–406.

262. R. Y. Qu, "Use of Oleanolic Acid for Human Hepatitis," *Guangzhou Medicine* 3 (1981): 41–43.

263. G. B. Singh et al., "Anti-Inflammatory Activity of Oleanolic Acid in Rats and Mice," *Journal of Pharmacy and Pharmacology* 44 (1992): 456–58. In addition to the actions noted in the main text, oleanolic acid has shown cholesterol-lowering and anti-ulcer activities. See J. Liu et al., "The Effects of 10 Triterpenoid Compounds on Experimental Liver Injury in Mice," *Fundamental and Applied Toxicology* 22 (1994): 34–40.

264. See note 223 above.

265. K. Umehara et al., "Studies on Differentiation-Inducing Activities of Triterpenes," *Chemical and Pharmaceutical Bulletin* 40 (1992): 401–5.

266. S. J. Collins et al., "Continuous Frowth and Differentiation of Human Myeloid Leukeamic Cells in Suspension Culture," *Nature* 270 (1977): 347–49.

267. See note 265 above.

268. K. Umehara et al., "Studies on Differentiation-Inducers from Arctium Fructus," *Chemical and Pharmaceutical Bulletin* 41 (1993): 1774–79.

269. T. Kinoshita et al., "Induction of Differentiation in Murine Erythroleukemia Cells by Flavonoids," *Chemical and Pharmaceutical Bulletin* 33 (1985): 4109–12.

270. See note 244 above.

271. See note 269 above.

272. D. V. C. Awang et al., "Naphthoquinone Constituents of Commercial Lapacho/Pau d'Arco/Taheebo Products," *Journal of Herbs, Spices and Medicinal Plants* 2, no. 4 (1994), publication pending.

273. See notes 96 and 219 above.

274. Hinrich Möeller and Matthias Potokar, "Preparation of Alkoxybenzoates As Inflammation Inhibitors for Cosmetics and Topical Drugs," German Patent DE 38 37 969 A1, May 10, 1990.

275. See note 157 above.

276. See notes 96 and 219 above.

277. See note 96 above.

278. "Veratric Acid" in *Merck Index*, 11th ed. (Rahway, N.J.: Merck and Co., 1989), 1564.

279. Z. Suprynowicz et al., "Determination of Veratric Acid and Its Metabolites in Biological Material by Ion-Pair High Performance Liquid Chromatography," *Journal of Chromatography* 286 (1984): 253–60.

280. R. G. Dickinson et al., "Facile Hydrolysis of Mebeverine *In Vitro* and *In Vivo*: Negligible Circulating Concentrations of the Drug after Oral Administration," *Journal of Pharmaceutical Sciences* 80 (1991): 952–57.

281. P. S. Gupta et al., "A Musculotropic-Antispasmodic in Duodenal Ulcer," *British Journal of Clinical Practice* 26 (1972): 35–36.

282. C. Tasman-Jones, "Mebeverine in Patients with the Irritable Colon Syndrome: Double Blind Study," *New Zealand Medical Journal* 77 (1973): 232–35.

283. See note 89 above.

284. See note 280 above.

285. A. D. Hertog and J. V. D. Akker, "The Action of Mebeverine and Metabolites on Mammalian Non-Myelinated Nerve Fibres," *European Journal of Pharmacology* 139 (1987): 353–55.

286. G. M. Laekerman et al., "Eugenol and Analogues As Antiplatelet Compounds," *Planta Medica* 52 (1986): 431 (Poster K33).

287. See note 96 above.

288. See note 272 above.

289. P. J. Houghton et al., "The Constituents of Commercial Lapacho," *Journal of Pharmacy and Pharmacology* 44, suppl. (1992): 1081.

290. See note 272 above.

291. See note 289 above.

292. A. L. Bandoni et al., "Survey of Argentine Medicinal Plants. I. Folklore and Phytochemical Screening," *Lloydia* 35 (1972): 69–80.

293. P. Forgacs et al., "Études Phytochimiques et Activités Biologiques de 18 Plantes de la Guyane Française," *Plantes Médicinales et Phytothérapie* 17 (1983): 22–32.

294. C. Djerassi et al., "Terpenoids. XXII. Triterpenes from Some Mexican and South American Plants," *Journal of the American Chemical Society* 78 (1956): 2312–15.

295. See note 210 above.

296. O. Sticher, "Plant Mono, Di- and Sesquiterpenoids with Pharmacological or Therapeutical Activity," in *New Natural Products and Plant Drugs with Pharmacological, Biological, or Therapeutical Activity*, eds., H. Wagner and P. Wolff (Berlin: Springer-Verlag, 1977), 137–76. In mice, the terpenes of fennel, cloves, and eucalyptus increase the production of enzymes in the upper digestive tract that help the body to detoxify carcinogens. See L. K. T. Lam and B. Zheng, "Effects of Essential Oils on Glutathione *S*-Transferase Activity in Mice," *Journal of Agriculture and Food Chemistry* 39 (1991), 660–62.

297. C. H. Su et al., "Hepato-Protective Triterpenoids from *Ganoderma tsugae* Murrill," *Mushroom Biology and Mushroom Products*, eds., Shu-ting Chang et al., Proceedings of the First International Conference on Mushroom Biology and Mushroom Products, August 23–26, 1993, Chinese University of Hong Kong, Hong Kong. (Shatin, N.T., Hong Kong: Chinese University Press, 1993), 275–83.

298. Terry Willard and Kenneth Jones, *Reishi Mushroom: Herb of Spiritual Potency and Medical Wonder* (Seattle: Sylvan Press, 1990), 62–65, 136–39.

299. See note 46 above.

300. See note 96 above.

301. Gail Nielsen, Castro Valley, California; personal communication, November 1984.

302. See note 220 above.

303. Takuiji Nakamura et al., "Antitumor Agents Containing Saponins of Bignoniaceae," Japanese Patent 63–101329, May 6, 1988, 4 pp. (in Japanese).

304. See note 149 above.
305. R. Wasicky et al., "Fitoquímica de *Tabebuia* sp. ("Ipê Roxo"): I—Anaise de Alguns Princípios," *Revista de Faculdade Farmácia e Bioquímica da Universidad São Paulo* 5 (1967): 383–95.
306. See note 220 above.
307. See notes 6 and 305 above.
308. See note 11 above.
309. Octaviano Gaiarsa, "Relatório do Instituto Carlo Erba Realizado Pelos Profs. Sirtori, Tommasini e Douter Angelucci" (Santo André, State of São Paulo, Brazil, undated), 14 pp. Translation.
310. See notes 4, 6, and 17 above.
311. Marilda M. de Oliveira, Institute of Biology, São Paulo; letter to the author, January 9, 1985.
312. See note 16 above.
313. Varro E. Tyler, "Pau D'Arco (Taheebo) Herbal Tea," *California Council Against Health Fraud, Inc. Newsletter* 6, no. 5 (1983): 3.
314. See note 2 above.
315. See note 216 above.
316. Gentry, *Bignoniaceae—Part II,* 266–68.
317. See note 216 above.
318. See note 2 above.
319. P. Arenas and R. M. Azorero, "Plants of Common Use in Paraguayan Folk Medicine for Regulating Fertility," *Economic Botany* 31 (1977): 298–301.
320. Gentry, *Bignoniaceae—Part II,* 144–45.
321. See note 28 above.
322. Ibid.
323. Richard Evans Schultes; personal communication, October 27, 1993.
324. See note 293 above.
325. See note 216 above.
326. See note 1 above.
327. See note 19 above.
328. Teodoro Meyer, *Sodre Uso Tejido Cortical Vivo de Especies do Bignoniaceas,* undated. Translation.
329. Paul Martinez Crovetto, *Las Plantas Utilizadas en Medicina Popular en el Noroeste de Corrientes (Republica Argentina),* Miscelanea no. 69 (Tucuman, Argentina: Ministerio de Cultura y Educacion, Foundacion Miguel Lillo, 1981), 102. Translation.
330. See note 319 above.
331. See note 1 above.
332. Teodoro Meyer, *Lapachol-Meyer* (Tucuman, Argentina: Foundation Miguel Lillo, undated brochure). Translation.
333. J. F. Morton, "Tannin As a Carcinogen in Bush Tea: Tea, Maté, and Khat," in *Chemistry and Significance of Condensed Tannins,* eds., R.W. Hemingway and J. J. Karchesy (New York: Plenum Publishing, 1989), 403–16.
334. See note 305 above.

CHAPTER FIVE

1. Teodoro Meyer, Curriculum vitae.
2. Teodoro Meyer, "Progresso de los Estudios en el Campo de la Flora del Noroeste Argentino, desde 1937 hasta la Fecha," *Conference of the Ministry of Edu-*

    cation and Justice, Foundation Miguel Lillo, Tucuman, Argentina, October
    23, 1966.
3. Joao Meirelles Filho, "The Perils of Deforestation," *World Press Review* (May
    1985): 33.
4. Bob Levin and Moyra Ashford, "The Last Frontier," *MacLean's* (January 19,
    1987): 28.
5. R. Monastersky, "The Deforestation Debate," *Science News* 144 (July 10,
    1993): 26–27.
6. O. R. Gottlieb and W. B. Mors, "Potential Utilization of Brazilian Wood Ex-
    tractives," *Journal of Agricultural and Food Chemistry* 28 (1980): 196–215.
7. R. E. Schultes, "Gifts of the Amazon Flora to the World," *Arnoldia* 50 (1990):
    21–33.
8. "Commercial Potential of Medicinal Plants," *Scrip World Pharmaceutical News*,
    no. 1400 (April 1989): 31.
9. A. Bonati, "Medicinal Plants and Industry," *Journal of Ethnopharmacology* 2
    (1980): 167–71.
10. Alwyn H. Gentry; letter to Dr. Dennis Awang, December 18, 1987.
11. A. H. Gentry, "A Synopsis of Bignoniaceae Ethnobotany and Economic
    Botany," *Annals of the Missouri Botanical Garden* 79 (1992): 53–64.
12. Alwyn H. Gentry; letter to Dr. Dennis Awang, March 11, 1987.
13. See notes 10 and 11 above.
14. See note 11 above.
15. Peter T. White, "Tropical Rain Forests: Nature's Dwindling Treasures," *Na-
    tional Geographic* (January 1983): 2–9, 20–47.
16. Ibid.
17. Ronald Sullivan, "Theodore Parker, Alwyn Gentry, Biologists, Die in Airplane
    Crash," *The New York Times*, August 6, 1993, C16.
18. Sharon Begley, "Zombies and Other Mysteries: Ethnobotanists Seek Magical,
    Medicinal Plants," *Newsweek* (February 22, 1988): 79.
19. E. W. Davis, "The Ethnobotany of Chamairo: *Mussatia hyacinthina*," *Journal
    of Ethnopharmacology* 9 (1983): 225–36.
20. Luis Eduardo Luna, "Vegetalismo. Shamanism Among the Mestizo Popula-
    tion of the Peruvian Amazon." *Acta Universitatis Stockholmiensis* 27 (1986):
    40.
21. Ibid., 163–64.
22. Ibid., 29.
23. Ibid.
24. World Health Organization, *The Promotion and Development of Traditional
    Medicine*, Technical Report Series 622 (Geneva, Switzerland: World Health
    Organization, 1978), 15.
25. E. Elizabetsky, "New Directions in Ethnopharmacology," *Journal of
    Ethnobiology* 6 (1986): 121–28.
26. Joseph W. Bastien, *Drum and Stethoscope. Integrating Ethnomedicine and
    Biomedicine in Bolivia* (Salt Lake City: University of Utah Press, 1992): 57,99.
27. Joseph W. Bastien, *Healers of the Andes* (Salt Lake City: University of Utah
    Press, 1987), 86–93.
28. N. R. Farnsworth, "The Development of Pharmacological and Chemical Re-
    search for Application to Traditional Medicine in Developing Countries," *Jour-
    nal of Ethnopharmacology* 2 (1980): 173–81.

29. P. Bennett, "Nicole Maxwell: The Witch Doctor's Apprentice," *International Wildlife* (May/June 1984): 22–23.
30. V. Morell, "Jungle Prescriptions," *International Wildlife* (May/June 1984): 18, 23, 24.
31. N. Maxwell, "Jungle Pharmacy," *South American Explorer* 1 (1979): 8–13.
32. See note 30 above.
33. N. R. Farnsworth, "How Can the Well Be Dry When It Is Filled With Water," *Economic Botany* 38 (1984): 4–9.
34. D. D. Soejarto and N. R. Farnsworth, "Tropical Rainforests: Potential Sources of New Drugs?" *Perspectives in Biology and Medicine* 32 (1989): 244–56.
35. Norman R. Farnsworth and Djaja D. Soejarto, "Global Importance of Medicinal Plants," in *The Conservation of Medicinal Plants*, eds., Olayiwola Akerele et al. (Cambridge, England: Cambridge University Press, 1991), 25–42.
36. See notes 33 and 34 above.
37. R. W. Spjut, "Limitations of a Random Screen: Search for New Anticancer Drugs in Higher Plants," *Economic Botany* 39 (1985): 266–88.
38. See note 30 above.
39. See note 26 above.
40. See notes 26 and 33–37 above.
41. R. W. Spjut and R. E. Perdue, Jr., "Plant Folklore: A Tool for Predicting Sources of Antitumor Activity?" *Cancer Treatment Reports* 60 (1976): 979–85.
42. N. R. Farnsworth and C. J. Kaas, "An Approach Utilizing Information from Traditional Medicine to Identify Tumor-Inhibiting Plants," *Journal of Ethnopharmacology* 3 (1981): 85–99.
43. G. Penso, "The Role of WHO in the Selection and Characterization of Medicinal Plants (Vegetable Drugs)," *Journal of Ethnopharmacology* 2 (1980): 183–88.
44. E. S. Ayensu, "The Healing Plants," *Unasylva* 35 (1983): 2–6.
45. World Health Organization, *Promotion and Development*, 13–14.
46. Norman Macrae, "Reducing Medical Costs," *World Press Review* (July 1984): 27–29.
47. See note 25 above.
48. T. Catsambas and S. Foster, "Spending Money Sensibly: The Case of Essential Drugs," *Finance and Development* 23 (December 1986): 29–32.
49. M. F. Balandrin et al., "Natural Plant Chemicals: Sources of Industrial and Medicinal Materials," *Science* 228 (1985): 1154–60.
50. See note 33 above.

INDEX